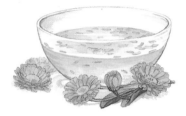

HEALTH AND HEALING
THE NATURAL WAY

NATURAL
REMEDIES

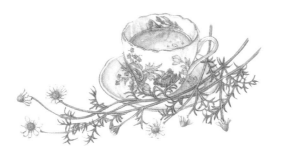

HEALTH AND HEALING
THE NATURAL WAY

NATURAL
REMEDIES

PUBLISHED BY

THE READER'S DIGEST ASSOCIATION, INC.

PLEASANTVILLE, NEW YORK/ MONTREAL

A READER'S DIGEST BOOK
Produced by
Carroll & Brown Limited, London

CARROLL & BROWN

Managing Editor Denis Kennedy
Art Director Chrissie Lloyd

Series Editor Arlene Sobel
Series Art Editor Johnny Pau

Editor Kesta Desmond
Assistant Editor Laura Price

Art Editor Carmel O'Neill
Designer Gemma Pearl

Photographers David Murray, Jules Selmes, Ian Boddy

Production Lorraine Baird, Wendy Rogers,
Amanda Mackie

Computer Management John Clifford, Caroline Turner

CONSULTANTS AND CONTRIBUTORS

Richard Adams, Dip. Phyt.
Member of the National Institute of Medical Herbalists

Helen Barnett, B.Pharm., Lic.Ac., M.B.Ac.A.
Chinese herbalist, acupuncturist, pharmacist

Susanna Dowie, Lic.Ac., M.T.Ac.S., R.W.T.A.
*Licentiate in Acupuncture and Chinese Medicine
Member of the Traditional Acupuncture Society*

Prof. Edzard Ernst
*Chair in Complementary Medicine
Postgraduate Medical School
University of Exeter*

Dr. Lesley Hickin,
M.B., B.S., B.Sc., D.R.C.O.G., M.R.C.G.P.
General Practitioner

Melanie Hulse, L.M.T.
Licensed Massage Therapist

Roger Newman Turner, B.Ac., N.D., D.O.
*Member of the Register of Naturopaths
Member of the Register of Osteopaths*

WRITERS

Anita Bean, B.Sc., Anthony Hillin, B.S.S., C.Q.S.W., Anne
Hooper, Siobhan McGee, T.I.D.H.A., R.Q.A., Michael
MacIntyre, M.A., M.N.I.M.H., M.R.T.C.M., Robin Munro,
Ph.D., Dee Pilgrim, Jerome Whitney, B.Sc., M.Sc., M.A.

MEDICAL ILLUSTRATIONS CONSULTANT

Dr. Frances Williams, M.B., B.Chir.,
M.R.C.P., D.T.M.&H.

READER'S DIGEST PROJECT STAFF

Series Editor Gayla Visalli
Project Editor Christine Morgan
Senior Associate Art Editor Nancy Mace
Editorial Director, Health & Medicine Wayne Kalyn
Associate Designer Jennifer R. Tokarski
Production Technology Manager Douglas A. Croll
Editorial Manager Christine R. Guido

READER'S DIGEST ILLUSTRATED REFERENCE BOOKS, U.S.

Editor-in-Chief Christopher Cavanaugh
Art Director Joan Mazzeo
Operations Manager William J. Cassidy

Address any comments about *Natural Remedies* to
Reader's Digest, Editor-in-Chief, U.S. Illustrated Reference Books,
Reader's Digest Road, Pleasantville, NY 10570

You can also visit us on the World Wide Web at:
www.readersdigest.com

To order additional copies of *Natural Remedies*,
call 1-800-846-2100

Library of Congress Cataloging in Publication Data

Natural remedies.
     p.   cm. — (Health and healing the natural way)
Includes index.
ISBN 0-89577-834-3
     1. Naturopathy. I. Reader's Digest Association. II. Series.
RZ440.N36 1995
615.5—dc20   95-20225

Reader's Digest and the Pegasus logo are registered trademarks of
The Reader's Digest Association, Inc.
Printed in the United States of America
Third Printing, January 2001

The information in this book is for reference only: It is not
intended as a substitute for a physician's diagnosis and care. The
editors urge anyone with continuing medical problems or
symptoms to consult a qualified physician.

FOREWORD

Since the late 19th century conventional medical treatment has been considered the first—and often only—health-care option for people living in the West. In recent years, however, alternative therapies, some of them based on healing techniques thousands of years old, have taken their place alongside orthodox medicine, and proved to be of inestimable value to the health of many who use a natural approach to health care. Nevertheless, the recognition and respect accorded to natural medicine is still somewhat limited, for the simple reason that the therapies remain unfamiliar to many people.

The goal of NATURAL REMEDIES is to introduce readers to therapies that can help them prevent illness and achieve and maintain good health and a sense of well-being. In addition to promoting the benefits of a healthy diet and exercise, the book covers a wide range of treatments, from acupuncture to aromatherapy, herbal medicine to hydrotherapy, reflexology to Rolfing, and much more.

It first explains individual therapies and introduces the techniques used by their practitioners. Successive chapters focus on different disorders and problems—physical and emotional—that can be treated both conventionally and with one or more natural therapies. To illuminate these therapies further, special sections are devoted to the work of various practitioners, explaining what is done during a typical session with one and what you can do at home. Plus there are case studies that reveal how people have used natural remedies to alleviate symptoms and maintain good health and many step-by-step illustrations that guide you through treatments, making them more accessible.

NATURAL REMEDIES shows you how to restore and enrich your health with good care and an understanding of what you can do to help your body heal itself.

CONTENTS

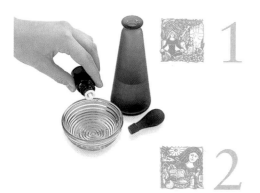

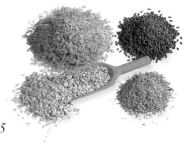

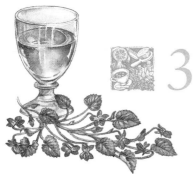

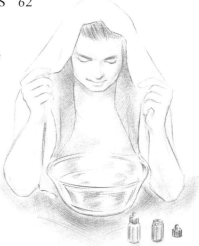

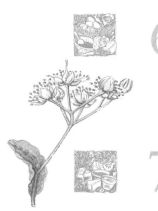

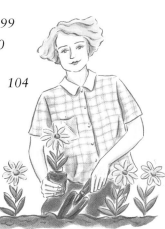

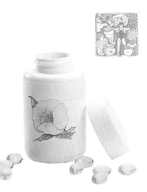
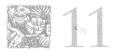

NATURAL HEALING

As the barriers between conventional and natural medicine are broken down, health care is widening to encompass a revised view of the healer and the healed.

YEHUDI MENUHIN
The internationally acclaimed violinist Yehudi Menuhin is a great proponent of natural therapies. He regularly practices yoga as a way of keeping supple and mentally calm.

HERBALISM
Many plants have medicinal properties. Herbalists use these plants to treat the symptoms of illness or to bolster the body's natural immunity.

One of the most important trends in medicine in recent years has been the increased responsibility people are taking for their own health. The days are disappearing when people had little knowledge of the workings of their bodies and believed that every complaint could be cured by a prescription from a doctor or, failing that, an operation. Now many recognize that they can influence their own health and well-being by paying attention to what foods they eat, how much they exercise, how they manage stress, and how they care for themselves when they are ill. Natural medicine offers an impressive array of resources to help us take good care of our health, and as more is learned about these natural healing techniques, they are becoming an increasingly popular way of preventing and treating many acute and chronic ailments. In fact, recent surveys indicate that one-third of all North Americans have already tried at least one natural therapy.

Most of the natural remedies described in this book are derived from age-old healing techniques. Rather than replacing the need for conventional medical care, they are recommended here as options that can be used in conjunction with orthodox treatment.

WHY NATURAL REMEDIES?

There has never been a greater demand for natural remedies, as increasingly people search for treatments that are effective yet safe. Fears about the harmful side effects of some prescription drugs, for example, are prompting people to seek alternatives. Moreover, today's high-tech medicine, with its surgical procedures that treat a specific part of the individual, has led many people to resent the impersonal nature of their health care and desire treatment that takes into account the whole person. They may also be prompted by the realization that conventional medicine may not cure many of the most common ailments, such as back pain, insomnia, headache, and depression. Nevertheless, there are situations when the powerful drugs and technological innovations of modern medicine are necessary and life-saving. Rapid, reliable measures are sometimes needed when our innate healing powers are facing tremendous odds. Luckily for most of us, serious accidents, injuries, and diseases are relatively rare, and our bodies, if left alone, are able to cope with most minor ailments and injuries. Hence the main emphasis in this book is on treatments that promote the body's own self-healing process.

Many plants contain active compounds that are as strong as those found in any modern drug, but they also contain other chemicals that modify the dominant compounds' effects, thus making some herbal remedies gentler and less toxic than prescription drugs when used as directed. Bach flower and homeopathic remedies are used in such infinitesimal dilutions that they are considered almost harmless at the potencies normally available.

Other natural therapies involve the use of water—bathing and compresses, for example—or vitamin and mineral supplements and dietary changes. Physical therapies like massage, reflexology, and acupressure can be done generally without risk. In many cases, the treatments are simple, relatively inexpensive, and they can be practiced in your home, although some require the skills of a professional practitioner.

FLOWERS, LEAVES, AND BERRIES
Herbal remedies may be made from any part of a plant. Active compounds are present in the flowers or leaves, stems or berries, bark or roots.

TREATING THE WHOLE PERSON

Approaching a patient as an individual—rather than as a collection of separate body parts—is the hallmark of holistic medicine. Holistic, or whole person, medicine recognizes that your health is dependent on the interaction of body and mind, and that to restore good health it is very important to consider both emotional and physical symptoms. For example, rather than merely suppressing symptoms of heartburn or indigestion with antacid or gas-reducing medications, holistic treatment may be directed at adjusting diet and eating patterns, managing stress, and identifying possible emotional problems.

As diverse as they are, all natural therapies are united by this holistic principle. In other words, when making a diagnosis, a practitioner will consider not only the immediate physical symptoms of an illness but also the overall health and physical resilience of the individual, his or her personality, behavior, lifestyle, and emotional state.

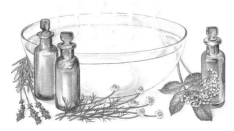

AROMATHERAPY
The essential oils used in aromatherapy are derived from herbs and other aromatic plants and trees. There are many ways of using them therapeutically. One popular method is to add them to a bowl of hot water and inhale the vapors. Another is to dilute them with a base oil and massage them into the skin.

YOGA POSES
Practicing yoga regularly has many benefits. It not only keeps your body flexible, but it is also an excellent method of relieving stress and promoting relaxation.

ANCIENT WISDOM, MODERN SKILLS

Many natural therapies can be traced through their evolution from ancient healing traditions. Others, however, are the result of the inspiration, innovation, and dedication of healers from all around the globe, who have developed, nurtured, and honed their skills based on their faith in the body's natural healing power and in the healing properties of the natural world.

Herbal remedies and acupuncture can be traced back thousands of years, while homeopathy and osteopathy were developed within the past 200 years. Rolfing, zone therapy, and reflexology are modern developments of the massage and reflex zone treatments known to the ancient Egyptians, Chinese, and Indians.

Regardless of a therapy's origins, natural practitioners assert that it should assist the body in healing itself and alleviating symptoms in ways that are in harmony with the body's normal responses.

BROADENING YOUR CHOICE

According to natural medicine practitioners, many healing processes can be enhanced using alternative therapies, and may even eliminate the need for more aggressive treatment prescribed by orthodox physicians. Natural preventive measures are perhaps the most effective of all. Simply by sticking to a well-balanced diet and exercising regularly, you can help ensure that your immune system is strong enough to resist illness and infection in the first place.

Even if you are taking prescribed medication or undergoing other more intensive medical treatment, it may still be possible to benefit from natural therapies. Massage, yoga, creative visualization, and reflexology, for example, will not conflict with most conventional medical care, although in some cases, the stronger prescription drugs might neutralize the benefits of certain natural medicinals, like homeopathic and herbal remedies. If you are receiving treatment from your doctor and you are in any doubt about how natural therapies can be used, ask him for advice.

In many respects, the worldwide influence of natural medicine has encouraged some orthodox physicians to reevaluate natural approaches to healing. There are indications that doctors are becoming more open to natural therapies, some of which were once a part of standard medical practice before the days of synthetic drugs and high-tech surgery. For example, conventional medicine has rediscovered the importance of nutrition in the management of certain illnesses, and doctors and hospitals now support women who opt for natural childbirth methods instead of anesthesia or painkilling drugs. This renewed interest and growing acceptance of natural therapies has prompted governmental as well as private support for scientific research into the merits of natural medicine therapies. Also, managed-care insurance companies are acknowledging the benefits of certain alternative approaches by reimbursing their costs.

WHEN TO USE NATURAL REMEDIES

Natural remedies are suitable for many acute and chronic illnesses, either as first-aid measures or as supportive treatment in conjunction with other medical care. Many remedies call for readily available tools and substances, such as your hands (for massage and acupressure), sheets, towels, and water (for hydrotherapy), and plants from the garden and herbs from the kitchen (for herbalism).

The best initial approach for minor acute conditions, such as colds, coughs, constipation, indigestion, diarrhea, rashes, and headaches, often is a natural remedy. Relief is usually prompt, and the worst of the disorder can be over in two or three days. If symptoms persist after using natural therapies or if they recur with undue frequency, you should see your doctor.

You may also achieve success in relieving the symptoms of chronic disorders such as arthritis, allergies, and migraines by using natural remedies. There is evidence, too, of the value of natural approaches in helping to prevent or aid in recovery from serious disorders such as heart disease. Indeed, many recent studies have suggested that certain lifestyle changes, like adopting a low-fat diet, getting regular exercise, and effectively managing stress, can help prevent and may even reverse coronary artery disease, as well as reduce the need for conventional drugs or surgery.

CHOOSING YOUR TREATMENT

To help you find a remedy for your particular problem, this book is divided into chapters dealing with different parts of the body and their common disorders. There are also chapters aimed at coping with health problems that affect men and women specifically or problems of an emotional nature. Several therapies are recommended for each complaint—some of them are preventive, some offer quick relief from the pressing discomfort of symptoms, and a number of them

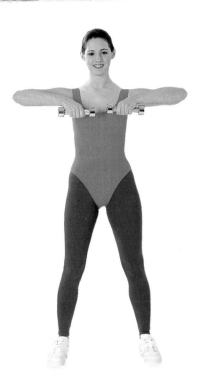

STRENGTH-TRAINING EXERCISE
Exercising with weights is an easy and effective way to build muscle, increase strength, and reduce your risk for many types of injuries.

EATING FOR HEALTH
To maintain good health, your body needs a daily supply of nutrients, particularly vitamins and minerals. A diet that is rich in raw fruits and vegetables is recommended by naturopaths to prevent many types of illness.

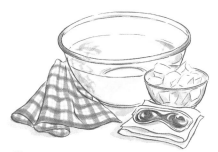

HYDROTHERAPY
Water is the most readily available natural remedy, yet its therapeutic value is often underestimated. Hydrotherapy offers a wide range of techniques to prevent and treat illness.

BACH FLOWER REMEDIES
Dr. Edward Bach identified 38 flower remedies to treat an array of emotional problems. Available in bottled form, a few drops of each remedy may be taken with water or in some cases dropped directly onto the tongue.

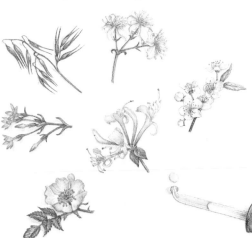

offer long-term solutions to illness. While some remedies can be prepared or practiced at home, others need to be purchased from a health food store or require a visit to a practitioner. Choose the treatment that is most convenient and appropriate to your symptoms, whether it is immediate help for a bee sting or long-term dietary treatment for a digestive disorder. Sometimes you may need to combine two or three treatments. With earache, for example, acupressure might relieve the pain, but you may also want to follow naturopathic dietary recommendations to reduce the inflammation that causes it and take a suitable homeopathic remedy to foster the drainage of the middle ear.

For certain complaints it may be necessary to obtain the help of a professional practitioner in addition to practicing self-help measures. Back pain, for example, may be relieved by massage and hydrotherapy at home, but you may also require treatment from an osteopath or chiropractor to rectify a misalignment of the muscles or vertebrae, which may be responsible for the problem.

GETTING PROFESSIONAL HELP

Most practitioners of natural therapies work in private practice, although some physicians now include practitioners like massage therapists and dietitians in their group practices. Doctors sometimes refer their patients to practitioners of natural medicine for specialized treatment such as acupuncture, hydrotherapy, osteopathy, and chiropractic. Many medical referrals are for problems involving the muscles and joints and stress-related conditions, but patients are also sent for help with other problems ranging from allergies to digestive troubles, skin disorders, and insomnia.

Government regulation of natural medicine practitioners varies from one state or province to another. Many people have received extensive training from specialized schools and belong to professional organizations that set standards and certify qualifications. When choosing a practitioner of natural medicine, the best advice is to be guided by a personal recommendation, if possible, and to ascertain if this person belongs to a professional organization. Many such groups can also provide you with a list of qualified practitioners in your area.

VISITING THE PRACTITIONER

When you visit a natural medicine practitioner, the first part of the consultation will be a discussion of your current symptoms, when they started, whether they are continuous or intermittent, and whether they are exacerbated by any particular activity. The practitioner will then build a picture of your medical history by asking questions about previous illnesses and those of your family. You are also likely to be asked about your eating and sleeping patterns, and some practitioners will ask about your emotional health, your relationships, and your lifestyle. Although some of this information may seem irrelevant to your symptoms, the practitioner must gain an overview of you as a person in order to decide upon the most appropriate remedy.

The second part of a consultation may consist of a physical examination. The type of examination will depend on the particular therapy you have chosen. For instance, a Chinese herbalist will take your pulse at three different positions on each wrist and look at the color and texture of your tongue. A chiropractor will feel your spine to find irregularities or areas of tenderness and he or she may also decide to take X-rays. A homeopath will take your blood pressure and pulse at rest, in the same way a conventional medical doctor would.

The first visit to a natural practitioner may be quite lengthy (the average initial natural medical consultation is six times longer than a consultation with a conventional doctor). Subsequent visits are likely to be follow-ups—you may find that these sessions are much shorter. In the case of exercises like yoga or tai chi, you will learn new poses or movements as well as practice those you have been taught. The number of visits you need with a practitioner depends on the severity of your illness and whether your condition is acute or chronic. One survey in the United States found that people who were receiving natural treatments made an average of 19 visits in the course of a year.

Keep in mind that while the therapies described in this book are normally very safe, even natural remedies can have dangerous side effects if used excessively or inappropriately. Also, even when used properly, herbal preparations can trigger allergic reactions in some people. And in some cases, such as with many homeopathic remedies, treatment may cause symptoms to become temporarily more acute; this effect should be short-lived. If you are in any doubt about your ailment or symptoms, you should always seek advice from your doctor.

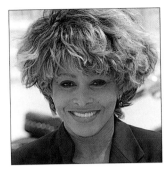

TINA TURNER
Rock star Tina Turner uses homeopathic remedies to maintain health and alleviate the symptoms of illness.

ACUPUNCTURE
Inserting fine needles into specific points on the body is believed to regulate the flow of energy, or chi, thus enabling the body to cure itself of illness.

WHEN SHOULD YOU SEE YOUR DOCTOR?

When you are ill you should always obtain a doctor's diagnosis first. This is particularly important if you answer yes to any of the questions below, since these symptoms are likely to require conventional treatment, and natural remedies may be ineffective or inappropriate. In other cases, if you try natural remedies and your symptoms worsen or fail to improve, you should see your doctor.

Q **ARE YOU SUFFERING FROM SEVERE HEAD, CHEST, OR ABDOMINAL PAIN?**
Sudden and severe pain in the head may be a sign of meningitis, especially if accompanied by fever, vomiting, oversensitivity to light, and a stiff neck. Pain in the abdomen could indicate appendicitis or internal bleeding, whereas chest pain may be due to angina. It is important that your doctor diagnose and treat these serious conditions.

Q **IS IT DIFFICULT TO BREATHE OR SWALLOW?**
Any obstruction, swelling, or narrowing of the airways or throat that makes it difficult to swallow or impedes breathing should receive immediate medical attention.

Q **ARE YOUR LEGS SWOLLEN?**
Swelling of either the legs or feet, particularly when accompanied by pain or tenderness of the calves that is not the consequence of an injury, could indicate a serious circulatory disorder.

Q **HAVE YOU BEEN SUFFERING FROM PAIN OR FEVER FOR MORE THAN 24 HOURS?**
Any symptoms of pain, inflammation, or fever that do not improve after 24 hours of natural remedies should receive a conventional medical assessment. You may have developed a serious disorder or there may be secondary problems that will not respond to natural medicine.

Q **DO YOU HAVE A HISTORY OF A SERIOUS CHRONIC CONDITION—HEART DISEASE OR EPILEPSY, FOR EXAMPLE?**
Cardiovascular, circulatory, and neurological disorders may be exacerbated by some therapies, especially those employing movement, manipulation, heat treatment, or certain herbs.

ESSENTIAL OILS
Since essential oils contain the volatile constituents of plants in a highly concentrated form, they should be stored and used with care. Always keep oils in dark glass bottles.

CHAPTER 1

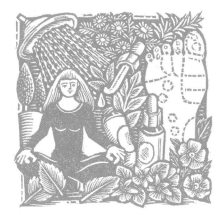

THE THERAPIES

The choice of natural therapies available today—whether traditional or innovative, Eastern or Western—is wider than ever. They range from herbalism and homeopathy to manipulative therapies such as massage and chiropractic to the mind-body techniques of biofeedback and hypnotherapy. What most natural therapies have in common is their holistic approach. Rather than treating an isolated symptom, they aim to improve the health of the whole body.

HEALING WITH NATURAL MEDICINALS

The medicinal and healing properties in plants, foods, and inorganic substances, such as mineral salts, can be harnessed and used as natural "drugs."

Some natural medicinals are used in their original or raw form. For instance, an easily recognizable herb such as rosemary can be picked from the garden and used to make an infusion. Other remedies are prepared from extracts of natural substances, which are available over the counter at pharmacies and health food stores. These include Bach flower remedies, essential oils, and homeopathic pills.

HERBALISM

Before the age of manufactured medicines, people used a great many plant remedies. Although a number of modern drugs are actually derived from plants, there has recently been a resurgence of interest in using herbs in their natural form, in the belief that they offer a relatively safe and effective alternative to pharmaceuticals.

When used as recommended, many herbal preparations are quite safe. However, as with anything you put in or on your body, you should have as much knowledge as possible and proceed with caution and common sense. Some herbs, comfrey for example, can be toxic if ingested, though it can safely be used in topical preparations applied to unbroken skin. Others can be dangerous for pregnant women, anyone suffering from a specific medical condition like high blood pressure, or a person taking other prescribed medications (drugs and herbs may interact, producing adverse effects). Still others may cause allergic reactions, especially in people who normally suffer from hay fever.

The herbs in this book are not considered toxic, and if there are contraindications to their use, these are mentioned. If you suffer any side effects, stop taking the remedy and consult a doctor or reputable herbalist.

Herbs can be taken in a variety of ways (see opposite page) and for many purposes. They may be used to eliminate toxins, stimulate the body's immune system, or tone the whole body. Among the range of disorders that respond well to herbal remedies are digestive complaints, skin problems, colds, insomnia, and arthritis.

The most effective remedies are likely to be those prepared for you by an herbalist. If you make your own preparations, consider buying standardized dried herbal products at a health food store or pharmacy. These have been processed in such a way that the producer can guarantee how much of the active ingredients are available, thus removing the guesswork that is part of harvesting your own plants or buying herbs in bulk.

Herbal preparations

The most common herbal preparations that can be made at home are infusions, decoctions, tinctures, poultices, and compresses.

An infusion is made in the same way as a pot of tea (herbal infusions are sometimes referred to as teas). For a standard infusion, place 1 ounce of a dried herb or 2½ ounces of a fresh herb in a glass or china teapot. If using several herbs, they should still add up to 1 ounce dried or 2 ounces fresh. Add 16 fluid ounces (2 cups) of boiling water; steep for 10 to 20 minutes. Strain the infusion through a fine sieve or piece of muslin and drink it hot. The standard dosage for an herbal infusion is 1 cup 3 times a day.

Decoctions are made instead of infusions when roots or the hard, woody parts of the plant are used. Because the active compounds are harder to extract, simply pouring boiling water onto the herb is not sufficient. Instead, the herbs are boiled in water and then strained. Unpleasant-tasting

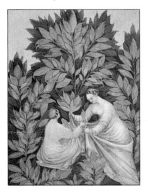

GATHERING HERBS
Picking and using freshly grown herbs for medicinal purposes is a practice that dates back through the ages. Here, two 15th-century women are shown gathering sage.

PREPARING HERBAL REMEDIES AT HOME

Both fresh and dried herbs can be used to make herbal remedies. (You will need a kitchen scale to weigh the specified amounts and, in general, will need twice as much of the fresh product as the dried.) Fresh herbs are more potent, but dried ones have the advantage of being available all year-round from herbalists and health food stores. If you do pick fresh herbs, make sure that you can accurately identify the plants, and use them right away for best results. When stored in airtight containers in a cool, dry place, dried leaves keep their potency for six or seven months; roots, bark, and seeds remain effective for up to three years.

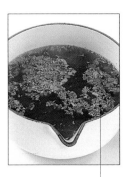
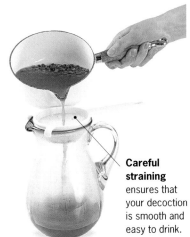
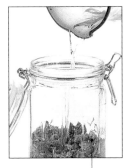
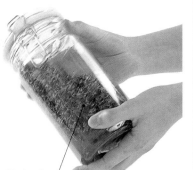

The woody parts of the herbs need lengthy boiling to release the active compounds.

Careful straining ensures that your decoction is smooth and easy to drink.

Keep the alcohol and herbs in an airtight container.

Shake the tincture regularly to ensure that the herbs and alcohol mix together.

MAKING A STANDARD DECOCTION
Place 1 ounce of the dried herb or 2 ounces of the fresh herb in 24 fluid ounces (3 cups) of water and bring to a boil. Allow to simmer for at least 20 minutes—an hour at most. Strain the decoction through a sieve while hot. If kept in a cool place, the decoction will last a day or two. The standard dosage is to take 1 cup 3 times a day.

MAKING A STANDARD TINCTURE
Take 2 cups of alcohol of at least 30 proof (vodka is suitable), and pour it over 4 ounces of dried herbs (8 ounces fresh). Keep the mixture in a warm place for two weeks, and shake daily. Strain the liquid through muslin into a dark, airtight bottle. Take 1 teaspoon 3 times a day. A tincture will last for at least a year.

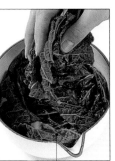
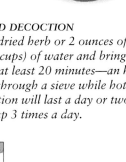
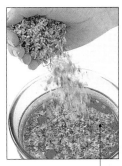
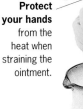
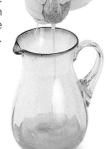

Fresh herbs need only brief, light boiling to prepare them for a poultice.

Wrap the hot boiled herbs around the affected area with strips of muslin.

Melt the petroleum jelly before adding the herbs.

Protect your hands from the heat when straining the ointment.

MAKING A POULTICE OR COMPRESS
Boil the herbs in a little water for 2 minutes (longer if the herbs are dried), then spread the mixture on strips of muslin and apply to the skin while hot. A compress is made in the same way, but instead of using the whole herb, a cloth dipped in an infusion or a decoction is used. Poultices and compresses should be as hot as is bearable when applied.

MAKING AN HERBAL OINTMENT
The simplest way to make an ointment is to simmer 2 tablespoons of a dried herb in 7 ounces of melted petroleum jelly for about 10 minutes. Stir well, then strain through fine gauze. While still hot, pour the liquid into a heat-proof container. Allow to cool, and seal the container. Ointments will keep usually for several weeks.

infusions or decoctions can be made more palatable with a little honey.

Although infusions and decoctions are usually taken internally, they can also be added to a bath or footbath, or used as a face wash or hair rinse (see page 59). You can add a standard infusion to bathwater by placing a small herb-filled tea infuser in the water, or by using an herbal bath bag. To make a bath bag, take a square piece of muslin, place a handful of herbs in the middle, then gather the corners and secure them with string. Attach the bag to your bathtub faucet so that the hot water runs through it.

An herbal tincture, which contains the active compound of an herb dissolved in alcohol, is also taken internally. Some people prefer tinctures to either infusions or decoctions because they are more palatable, they are quick and easy to use, and they keep longer. A tincture can be taken as is, or it may be diluted with a little water.

Compresses and poultices are used to apply herbs externally. These preparations are commonly employed to treat headaches, fevers, colds, and skin problems. You can seal in the heat of a compress or poultice by placing a layer of plastic wrap over the cloth after it has been applied to the skin. Alternatively, lay a hot water bottle over the compress or poultice.

Ointments are another topical use of herbs. An herbal ointment forms a protective, healing layer on the skin and can be used for a beauty treatment as well as for treating a skin problem.

When buying herbs, it is important to purchase the correct ones. The best way to ensure this is to ask for an herb by its Latin name; some, such as echinacea are actually better known by the Latin term. The chart below gives common names and Latin names for all the herbs mentioned in this book.

HOMEOPATHY

The principle that "like may be cured by like" is a cornerstone of homeopathy. Remedies are given that, if applied in the appro-

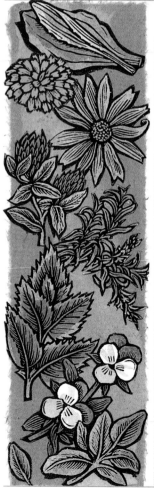

HERBS—COMMON AND LATIN NAMES

COMMON NAME	LATIN NAME	COMMON NAME	LATIN NAME
Aloe vera	Aloe vera	Cloves	Syzygium aromaticum
American cranesbill	Geranium maculatum	Collinsonia/Gravel root	Collinsonia canadensis
Angelica	Angelica archangelica	Cornsilk	Zea mays
Aniseed	Pimpinella anisum	Couchgrass	Elymus repens
Arnica	Arnica montana	Crampbark	Viburnum opulus
Basil	Ocimum basilicum	Cumin	Cuminum cyminum
Beth root	Trillium erectum	Damiana	Turnera diffusa
Black cohosh	Cimicifuga racemosa	Dandelion	Taraxacum officinale
Black horehound	Ballota nigra	Dill	Anethum graveolens
Blue cohosh	Caulophyllum thalictroides	Elder	Sambucus nigra
Bogbean	Menyanthes trifoliata	Elecampane	Inula helenium
Boneset	Eupatorium perfoliatum	Evening primrose	Oenothera biennis
Bucco/Buchu	Barosma betulina	Eucalyptus	Eucalyptus globulus
Buckthorn	Rhamnus frangula	False unicorn root	Chamaelirium luteum
Burdock	Arctium lappa	Fennel	Foeniculum officinale
Cardamom	Elettaria cardamomum	Fenugreek	Trigonella foenum-graecum
Cascara sagrada	Rhamnus purshiana	Feverfew	Tanacetum parthenium
Cayenne	Capsicum frutescens	Flax/Linseed	Linum usitatissimum
Celery	Apium graveolens	Garlic	Allium sativum
Chamomile	Matricaria recutita	Geranium	Pelargonium odorantissimum
Chaste berry	Vitex agnus-castus	Ginger	Zingiber officinalis
Chickweed	Stellaria media	Ginseng	Panax ginseng
Chinese angelica	Angelica sinensis	Goat's rue	Galega officinalis
Cinnamon	Cinnamomum zeylanicum	Goldenrod	Solidago virgaurea
Cleavers	Galium aparine	Goldenseal	Hydrastis canadensis

riate concentration, would produce in a healthy person symptoms similar to those of the disease being treated. The remedies are thought to accelerate the body's natural healing process. In contrast, conventional Western (allopathic) medicine seeks to eliminate the cause of the illness by destroying pathogens or excising diseased tissue.

Homeopathy was founded by the German physician, Dr. Samuel Hahnemann (1755–1843), who published his first paper on the subject in 1796. Intrigued by the use of cinchona (the natural source of quinine) in the treatment of malaria, he took a dose and discovered it produced shivering, sweating, and fever—the classic malaria symptoms. Hahnemann deduced that the symptoms of a disease were part of the body's healing mechanism, and by giving medicine that produced the same symptoms, recovery could be advanced. He went on to test arsenic, belladonna, and mercury on himself, and by observing the symptoms each of these substances produced, he was able to match them to specific illnesses. Additional tests seemed to confirm that a remedy would help to cure a condition with which it shared symptoms. The validity of this theory is still disputed, but homeopaths believe that their remedies provoke the body's natural healing mechanisms into overcoming the disease. They also believe that the more dilute the remedy, the more effective it is.

Homeopathic remedies come in the form of a pill to be dissolved under the tongue or a liquid to be dropped onto the tongue. Potencies are usually expressed by the centesimal system where one drop of a remedy is added to 99 drops of diluent (usually pure alcohol or water), producing a strength of 1c. One drop of this dilution is then further diluted in 99 drops of diluent to produce a strength of 2c and so on. However, a "high potency" remedy can be over 24c, meaning this process has been repeated 24 times.

The sources of homeopathic remedies are diverse. Some, such as pulsatilla, are produced from plants; others, such as silica, are

HERBS—COMMON AND LATIN NAMES

COMMON NAME	LATIN NAME	COMMON NAME	LATIN NAME
Hawthorn	Crataegus oxyacantha	Psyllium	Plantago psyllium
Honeysuckle	Lonicera periclymenum	Purple coneflower	Echinacea angustifolia
Hops	Humulus lupulus	Raspberry	Rubus idaeus
Lavender	Lavandula angustifolia	Red clover	Trifolium pratense
Lemon balm	Melissa officinalis	Rosemary	Rosmarinus officinalis
Licorice	Glycyrrhiza glabra	Sage	Salvia officinalis
Linden	Tilia europaea	Saw palmetto	Serenoa repens
Maidenhair tree	Ginkgo biloba	Slippery elm	Ulmus fulva
Marigold	Calendula officinalis	Squaw vine	Mitchella repens
Marjoram	Origanum onites	St. John's wort	Hypericum perforatum
Marsh mallow	Althaea officinalis	Stinging nettle	Urtica dioica
Meadowsweet	Filipendula ulmaria	Tea tree	Melaleuca alternifolia
Mint	Mentha spp.	Thyme	Thymus vulgaris
Motherwort	Leonurus cardiaca	Tree of life	Thuja occidentalis
Mullein	Verbascum thapsus	Valerian	Valeriana officinalis
Myrrh	Commiphora molmol	White horehound	Marrubium vulgare
Oats	Avena sativa	Wild lettuce	Lactuca virosa
Parsley	Petroselinum crispum	Wild yam	Dioscorea villosa
Pasqueflower	Anemone pulsatilla	Witch hazel	Hamamelis virginiana
Passionflower	Passiflora incarnata	Wood betony	Stachys officinalis
Peppermint	Mentha x piperita	Yarrow	Achillea millefolium
Periwinkle	Vinca major	Yellow dock	Rumex crispus
Pilewort	Ranunculus ficaria		
Plantain	Plantago lanceolata		
Prickly ash	Zanthoxylum americanum		

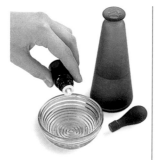

FRAGRANT MASSAGE OIL
Add your choice of an
essential oil to a base oil,
such as sweet almond oil,
and apply to the skin.

made from inorganic substances like rocks or mineral salts. A homeopath now has over 2,000 homeopathic remedies to select from and will make a selection only after having asked detailed questions about symptoms, diet, lifestyle, and even dental history. Homeopaths say that all these factors can affect the efficacy of the remedies. In fact, for every remedy there are thought to be three separate indications (reasons why the remedy may be appropriate). First, there are constitutional indications; this includes height, build, complexion, and stamina. Second, there are mental indications such as whether you are anxious or irritable. Third, there are the physical indications of your illness, for example, whether you have a headache or stomach pain.

Homeopathy is generally accepted as a gentle and safe therapy. Some homeopaths are also medical doctors and may prescribe homeopathic remedies in conjunction with conventional medical treatment.

Taking homeopathic remedies

If you decide to use homeopathy to treat your symptoms, it is wise to ask the advice of a qualified homeopath. Keep in mind, however, that homeopaths are not qualified to give a medical diagnosis. You can treat yourself at home using standard-strength over-the-counter pills. Although you will not harm yourself with these remedies, treatment is likely to be hit-and-miss without the expertise of the homeopath. You must follow certain homeopathic guidelines in order to achieve the most effective results.

Because the active constituent in homeopathic remedies has been very diluted it can easily become "polluted." Therefore, you are advised not to use the remedies while there is still the taste of food in your mouth, nor to eat for 20 minutes or so after taking a remedy. Strong-tasting substances such as coffee, mint, alcohol, tobacco, and spices may also reduce the potency of homeopathic remedies, so wait two hours after exposure to these items. You should also avoid handling the pills: take them by tipping them onto a teaspoon or into the bottle cap and placing them under your tongue.

Commonly used pills can be bought from pharmacists and health food stores at standard potencies—6c or 30c—and dosage instructions are given on the package. Although these remedies may initially exacerbate your symptoms they should quickly

alleviate them. If they do not, you may have selected the wrong treatment or you may be taking the remedy incorrectly. In this case you should seek the advice of a homeopath or see your doctor. If you are taking the wrong remedy, you will do yourself no harm because such extreme dilutions are used.

Since homeopathic pills contain lactose (a natural sugar in milk), you should avoid taking them if you are lactose intolerant. Ask a homeopath about remedies in liquid form.

Remedies should always be stored in a cool, dark place, and away from strong odors to avoid pollution.

FOLK MEDICINE

Folk medicine uses remedies made from plants and household items to treat illness. It is a healing tradition that has been passed down within families and communities from generation to generation. Although folk healing has long been ignored by conventional medicine, scientists are now finding real medical benefits to many of these simple remedies.

AROMATHERAPY

Using essential oils to alleviate both physical and emotional conditions is one of the most popular of all the natural therapies. Aromatherapy utilizes plant oils extracted by steam distillation or cold-pressing. Today, over 300 oils are used by practitioners.

Although touch, in the form of massage, is the main tool of the aromatherapist, there are many other ways of delivering essential oils to the nervous and circulatory systems of the body and olfactory center of the brain.

THE ANCIENT ART OF AROMATHERAPY
Egyptian stone carvings from around 600 B.C.
depict women collecting flowers to make
medicine or perfume.

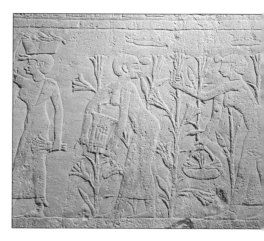

Oils can be added to a bath or footbath; inhaled from a bowl of steaming water; applied in lotions or compresses; used in a mouthwash; vaporized on an oil burner; and, very occasionally, applied directly to the skin or taken orally, although this is not advocated by all aromatherapists.

Sense of smell is a key component of aromatherapy. Although smell is probably the least appreciated of our senses, it is in fact extremely sensitive. Odors, both good and bad, can affect mood and behavior and can be used to have positive effects on emotional and physical health.

Research to validate aromatherapy is still incomplete, but aromatherapists say that the esters, aldehydes, and other chemicals the oils contain can have a powerful effect on our emotional state, relaxing us, energizing us, or relieving stress, anxiety, or depression. Essential oils may also relieve physical complaints. For example, lavender essential oil has been found to have analgesic properties and can be used to treat headaches, and tea tree oil is a proven antiviral, making it useful for cold sores and warts.

Using essential oils at home
Aromatherapy is a natural therapy that can be practiced quite easily at home. There are, however, some simple rules that you should apply for best results.
• Never apply undiluted oils to the skin—they are extremely concentrated and may cause irritation. The exception to this rule is tea tree essential oil.
• If you are pregnant, or if you suffer from high blood pressure, epilepsy, or skin allergies, you should consult a qualified aromatherapist before using essential oils.
• Essential oils should always be stored in dark, tightly sealed containers to keep them fresh and prevent evaporation. They should be kept out of the reach of children.

Inhalation
Inhaling essential oils simultaneously cleanses your skin, helps clear lung and sinus congestion, and eases sore throats. Add three drops of an essential oil to 2 cups of boiling water. Cover your head and the bowl with a small towel and inhale the vapors deeply and slowly. Repeat when necessary.

Massage
Mix your chosen essential oil with a carrier or base oil, such as sweet almond, jojoba, wheat germ, or peach kernel oil. Combine 20 to 25 drops of essential oil with 1/4 cup of the carrier oil (enough for a full-body massage). Warm your hands and apply the mixture to the skin with gentle massage strokes (see page 39).

Bathing
Three to four drops of an essential oil should be mixed with a small amount of baby shampoo and added to a hot bath. The oil is absorbed via inhalation and the pores of the skin. Essential oils can also be added to sponge baths, sitz baths, and footbaths.

Compresses
Fill a bowl with hot or cold water and add six drops of essential oil. Place a piece of soft cloth on the surface of the water so that it absorbs the oil. Wring out the excess water and apply the compress to the affected area. If the compress is hot, the heat can be retained by covering the cloth with plastic wrap or a hot water bottle.

Oil burners
Put a little water in the dish at the top of the burner and add three drops of an essential oil. Light the candle in the base of the burner and the oil's aroma will be released as it vaporizes over the heat. These burners are available in most health food stores.

HYDROTHERAPY
Using the healing properties of water is an ancient practice. If you consult a practitioner of hydrotherapy (naturopaths often use hydrotherapy techniques), you may be treated with sitz baths (you sit in hot water with your feet in cold water and then alternate), hot and cold compresses, alternating hot and cold baths, saunas, showers and steam baths, thalassatherapy (treatment with sea water), and whirlpools. Treatment with hot water increases circulation and

SITZ BATHS
A specially made sitz bath consists of a tub divided into two—one half is filled with hot water and the other cold. The person sits with hips in one half and feet in the other and then changes ends, moving the hips and feet alternately from hot to cold and back again in quick succession.

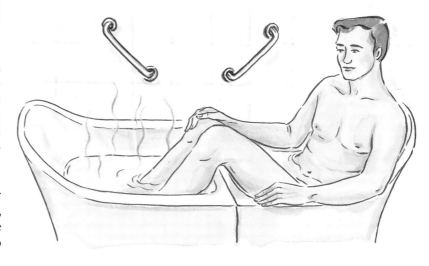

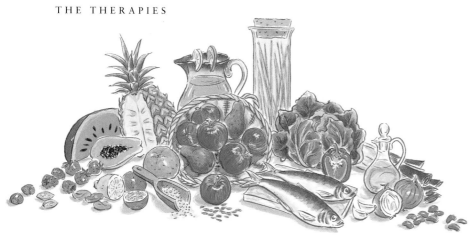

changes are central to naturopathy, practitioners are often trained in other treatments
such as herbalism and acupuncture.

The diagnostic procedures used by naturopaths include urine and blood tests, and, if
a naturopath cannot help, the patient will
be referred to an appropriate physician.

Although naturopathy has proved useful
in cases such as irritable bowel syndrome
and skin and joint problems, always have
symptoms checked by your doctor.

*FOODS TO IMPROVE
HEALTH
Naturopaths recommend
a diet that is high in fiber
and low in saturated fat.
Oily fish, which may
protect the heart, whole
grains, which are rich in
the B vitamins, and fruits
and vegetables will help
preserve health and
prevent illness.*

forces toxins from the body. Cold water
reduces swelling and inflammation.

The common practice in hydrotherapy of
applying alternating hot and cold water to the
body can stimulate the adrenal and endocrine
glands, reduce congestion, and also alleviate
inflammation due to tendinitis and arthritis,
and infections such as mastitis and urethritis.

Back pain, muscular strain, and sinus and
lung congestion are complaints that often
respond very well to hydrotherapy.

Using hydrotherapy techniques at home
Baths that have a shower attachment are
ideal for self-treatment. Try soaking for 15
minutes in a hot bath and then stand up and
take a quick cold shower to close the pores
of the skin and invigorate the body. The
whole process can be repeated for an even
greater effect, but you will not need to stay
in the hot water so long the second time.

The same principle can be applied to sitz
baths and footbaths—hot water is then
followed by a quick cold immersion. A sitz
bath—which would have to be specially
bought and installed in your home—enables
the hips and the feet to experience different
temperatures simultaneously, boosting the
circulation. See your doctor before trying
these treatments if you suffer from heart
disease or high blood pressure.

NATUROPATHY

The principle underlying naturopathy is
that the human body, given the right conditions, will cure itself of illness. Naturopaths
perceive some of the common causes of illness to be an unhealthy diet, inadequate
exercise, and an accumulation of waste
products in the body.

Remedies recommended by a naturopath
may include detoxification through fasting, elimination diets to identify possible
allergens, or simply eating more vitamin-
and mineral-rich foods. Although dietary

BACH FLOWER REMEDIES
Around the turn of the century, Dr. Edward
Bach (1880–1936), a British bacteriologist,
medical doctor, and homeopath, began to
experiment with flower remedies, using
them to treat certain emotional problems
including anxiety, depression, and anger.
He theorized that these plant remedies contained natural "vibrations" that could
restore harmony and health. Bach eventually devised 38 Bach flower remedies, ranging
from aspen to combat apprehension, to wild
rose for someone who is "stuck in a rut" and
making no effort to improve his situation.

One method involved in the preparation
of Bach flower remedies is floating the
flower heads in spring water in direct sunlight for three hours (this is to replicate
flower dew, which Bach believed to contain
medicinal properties). Another method
involves boiling the sprigs of the flowers or
catkins (this procedure is usually used for
the remedies that come from trees). The
remedies are then bottled in dark glass in
order to protect their potency.

A normal dosage is 2 drops of a remedy
combined with 1 fluid ounce (2 tablespoons)
of water; 4 drops of the resulting mixture are
taken orally 4 times a day. However, for
short-term problems, 2 drops of each remedy can be added to a glass of water to be
sipped throughout the day. You can also
mix the remedies together to treat specific
problems, but mixing more than five or six
is not considered necessary or appropriate.

In addition to the 38 Bach flower remedies—together with books and instructions
for their use—most health food stores now
stock Bach flower rescue remedy for use in
emotional "emergencies," such as sudden
shock or trauma. This is a combination of
several remedies. The Bach flower remedies
are not harmful and will not interfere with
other medical treatment.

*BACH FLOWER
REMEDIES
Some Bach flower
remedies, such as wild
rose, are prepared by
boiling the flowering
parts of a plant in pure
spring water. Wild rose is
recommended for apathy
and resignation.*

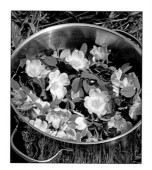

MOVEMENT AND MANIPULATION

Exercise and yoga movements are both strengthening and relaxing. Touch in the form of massage, manipulation, or pressure to specific points can help relax and heal the body.

Most movement and manipulation therapies involve being treated—or in the case of tai chi and yoga, taught—by a practitioner. The exceptions are exercise and massage that, providing you follow certain guidelines, you can learn and practice on your own.

EXERCISE

It is now recognized that any form of exercise, whether aerobic, strength, or flexibility exercise, can help prevent a range of both minor and serious illnesses. The many specific benefits of regular, moderate exercise include an increase in range of motion of the joints, and an improvement in bone density, muscle tone, cardiovascular fitness, and metabolic rate.

Exercise also stimulates the release of substances called endorphins. These are the body's natural painkillers and their release also promotes a feeling of well-being. This means that regular exercise can help you overcome emotional problems such as mild depression and anxiety.

Regular aerobic exercise, such as cycling or jogging, is particularly important for the prevention of heart disease—20 minutes of exercise three times a week in which the pulse rate reaches a target rate, determined by subtracting your age from 220. Any weight-bearing activity, like walking or aerobic exercise, for instance, will strengthen bones and help prevent osteoporosis.

Before you begin exercising, it is very important to warm up correctly (see page 86) to prevent muscle and joint injuries. You should seek medical advice before you exercise if you are overweight, unfit, or if you have a history of cardiovascular disease or other chronic illness.

YOGA

The purpose of the ancient Indian practice of yoga is to reunite the individual self (*jiva*) with pure consciousness or the absolute (Brahman). There are five components in yoga: relaxation; exercise (the yoga poses known as *asanas*); correct breathing (known as *pranayama* from *prana*, the Indian word for life force); a diet of wholesome foods; and mental self-discipline that is gained through meditation.

Some yoga poses, including the lotus position, can be traced back to 3000 B.C. Today, there are many different forms of yoga that you can practice. The main type taught in the West is Hatha yoga, a form that concentrates on correct breathing and movements to stretch and tone every muscle and joint in the body.

Practicing yoga helps relieve stress and maintain good health, and it may also strengthen the body's immune system. It is generally suitable for most people, but if you suffer from any condition involving chronic pain it is sensible to consult your doctor. Yoga may help counteract stiffness and pain in muscles, high blood pressure, asthma, and premenstrual syndrome. The majority of yoga teachers recommend practicing yoga daily in a comfortable, quiet environment. Do not force your body into a position that is difficult or very painful. If you find a movement uncomfortable, stop.

THE ALEXANDER TECHNIQUE

Australian actor, F. Matthias Alexander (1869–1955), developed this technique at the turn of the century after throat problems threatened his career. Using an arrangement of mirrors, he noticed that he constricted his throat muscles in such a way as to limit his

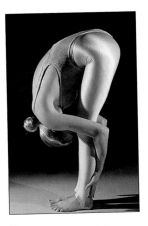

PRACTICING YOGA
The flexibility and muscular suppleness that can be achieved through practicing yoga will greatly increase the control you have over your body.

voice while performing, and that changing his posture not only caused his throat problems to disappear but also improved his overall health and mental well-being.

Alexander postulated that although children are born with freedom of movement, the subsequent stresses and strains of life cause them to draw their bodies into defensive postures, thus constricting the muscles of the neck and upper torso.

An Alexander technique teacher trains individuals to use their bodies in different ways, correcting the bad posture that leads to back pain and a stiff neck, easing joint strain, and strengthening the support of the internal organs. Sessions last 30 minutes to one hour and involve the teacher applying light manual pressure to make you aware of habitual problems of posture, for example, one hip higher than the other or a rounded spine. As sessions progress, the teacher will help you stand, sit, and crawl and gradually correct your posture.

You can apply what you have learned to your everyday activities from the very first lesson, but practitioners advocate a thorough mastering of the Alexander technique.

TAI CHI

More properly known as *tai chi chuan*, this ancient Chinese martial art is based on the belief that all life and material in the universe originated from a single source known as *tao*. *Chi*, or the life force, permeates tao and surrounds and flows through all human bodies in orderly patterns or lines that are called meridians.

When the flow of chi through a meridian becomes blocked or out of balance, illness will result. Therefore, in order to maintain good health, chi must be allowed to flow freely. It is believed that tai chi originated in

the 11th century when a man called Chang Senfeng developed a system of movements specifically to cultivate chi.

The movements of tai chi are gentle and should flow effortlessly into each other. This will promote the smooth flow of chi. It is best to take lessons from a fully trained tai chi teacher at first, since the postures or "forms" of tai chi are complicated. A short form consists of a series of 37 movements and will take between 5 and 10 minutes to perform, while a longer form consists of 108 movements and takes about 30 minutes.

Tai chi is widely recommended for relieving stress and anxiety, increasing flexibility, and toning muscles. It may also help to lower blood pressure.

OSTEOPATHY

According to osteopaths, many illnesses are caused by neuromusculoskeletal problems that can be treated with physical manipulation. Developed by an American, Dr. Andrew Taylor Still (1828–1917) in the late 19th century, osteopathy is based on his belief that when the body is correctly adjusted there is less strain on the musculoskeletal system. The result is that the body's other systems work more smoothly.

Through detailed questioning and feeling or palpating a patient's body, an osteopath attempts to discover why an illness has occurred. The problem may then be corrected by carefully manipulating the tissues, muscles, and joints. A series of more forceful manipulation movements are employed, including a "high velocity thrust," which can cause the joints to click. The treatment is usually agreeable rather than painful. Osteopathy is regularly used to treat cervical spondylosis, asthma, arthritis, and sports injuries. It is not recommended for people suffering from osteoporosis.

Osteopaths, or D.O.s, are now the most accepted of all the alternative health care practitioners and are fully qualified physicians. In America they are licensed to practice in all 50 states, and in Canada, in five of the provinces—Alberta, British Columbia, New Brunswick, Ontario, and Quebec. Just like M.D.s, osteopaths diagnose disease, prescribe drugs, refer patients to hospitals, and perform surgery. D.O.s are also represented in all of the practice specialties, including surgery, neurology, gynecology, obstetrics, and psychiatry.

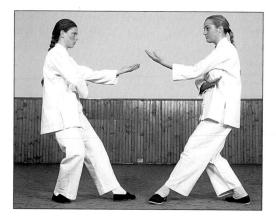

TAI CHI CHUAN
The highly focused and composed movements of tai chi can help you channel physical and emotional energy. As soon as the basic movements have been learned, you can begin to reap the benefits.

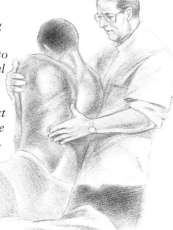

OSTEOPATHY
By manipulating the body, the osteopath aims to realign the spinal column and free any constricted nerves that affect the organs of the rest of the body.

Craniosacral therapy

Developed by William Garner Sutherland, who trained with Andrew Taylor Still, this branch of osteopathy applies osteopathic theory to the cranium. Garner believed that the misaligned bones of the skull could be coaxed back into normal working relationships using very gentle manipulation.

Craniosacral therapy is typically used for spinal and head injuries, including those to the face, mouth, and jaw. It is also used in babies and young children, whose cranial bones may have become misaligned at birth.

CHIROPRACTIC

Chiropractors use their hands to manipulate joints and vertebrae in order to restore the body to optimum health. Chiropractic was developed by a healer in Iowa, Daniel David Palmer (1845–1913), who believed that all disease is caused by vertebrae impinging on the spinal nerves. He came to this conclusion after he cured a local janitor's deafness by manipulating his spine.

Because the spine protects such a large part of the nervous system, if vertebrae become stiff or nerves become pinched or trapped, problems can occur almost anywhere in the body. The chiropractor's aim is to loosen up the stiffness in the spine and free the nerves, thereby removing the origin of physical disorders such as sciatica, slipped disks, arm and shoulder pain, lumbar pain, headaches, tennis elbow, leg and foot pain, and hand and wrist pain.

The first consultation with a chiropractor involves not only obtaining a detailed medical history, but often taking X-rays to locate the problem areas in the spine. Treatment typically involves removing the physical blockages in the spine that interfere with nerve function. Because spinal adjustments require precise movements, they should only be undertaken by a licensed chiropractor, and should not be given if the patient has osteoporosis, a spinal tumor, inflammation, or a recent bone fracture.

MASSAGE

All the civilizations of the ancient world used massage as a therapeutic remedy. Then, because of cultural taboos about the body and touching, massage fell out of favor in Europe until the 19th century, when a Swedish doctor, Per Hendrik Ling, developed the Swedish Movement Treatments. Swedish massage is still used today along with other types of massage, including acupuncture-based shiatsu—the application of pressure and massage to specific points.

There are sound physiological reasons why rubbing, kneading, and stroking various parts of the body should improve health. Moving muscles and soft tissues stimulates the circulation of blood and lymph, thus removing waste products and toxins from the area being massaged and supplying oxygen to the tissues.

A trained practitioner will not only be expert in the various massage strokes, like effleurage (long, sweeping movements), petrissage (kneading, wringing, or rolling movements), and tapotement (chopping movements with the side of the hand) but also will have knowledge of anatomy and physiology. Before the massage, a patient will be questioned about overall mental and physical health. Lotions, creams, or oils may be used in conjunction with massage strokes. Some massage therapists use essential oils diluted with a base oil during a massage. The oils are absorbed through the skin (see page 21).

Massage has proved useful for stress-related problems, arthritic conditions, muscular problems, back and neck pain, and sports injuries. Massage should not be undertaken by people taking anti-coagulant drugs because there is a risk of subcutaneous hemorrhage.

MASSAGE
The manipulation of the muscles through direct contact releases tension, leaving the patient relaxed and invigorated.

ROLFING

One of the most physical forms of body manipulation, Rolfing may be uncomfortable, even painful, both physically and emotionally for the patient. Devised by an American biochemist, Dr. Ida P. Rolf (1896–1976), this deep-tissue therapy uses a combination of vigorous massage and manipulation to release tension and to realign the body.

Rolf believed that the human body could be pushed out of alignment by the stresses of modern life. In order to remain functional, an individual would "fight" to keep the body in alignment, which drains it of energy, leaving it open to illness and pain.

To achieve realignment, a Rolfing practitioner may take photographs of a minimally clothed patient in order to detect any abnormal posture. The practitioner will then try to correct abnormalities by manipulating the patient's muscles and connective tissue using his or her knuckles, elbows, hands, and fingers.

ZONE THERAPY AND REFLEXOLOGY

Zone therapy was first introduced in the West in the early 20th century by American ear, nose, and throat specialist William H. Fitzgerald. He had discovered that pressure applied to certain parts of the nose caused numbness in areas of the face, and, as a result, mapped out other zones where this phenomenon occurred, coining the phrase "zone therapy." His studies were continued by Eunice Ingham, who believed that all parts of the body could be treated by applying pressure to the feet.

In reflexology, the body is thought to be divided into 10 vertical energy zones that run from the feet up through the body to the head and down through the arms to the hands. All the organs in a zone are connected by a flow of energy and the organs can be "accessed" by massaging specific areas on the hands and feet. Most reflexologists concentrate on the feet and claim to be able to diagnose a complaint by "reading" crystalline deposits in the area of the foot connected with the affected part of the body. The crystalline deposits are then broken down through the application of pressure and massage to the foot.

A consultation with a reflexologist will begin with the practitioner asking detailed questions about the person's general health and lifestyle, as well as an examination of the bare feet. Treatment involves firm pressure on specific areas of the feet (the pressure should never be painful). The number of sessions will vary depending on the problem. Practitioners say that gastrointestinal problems, heartburn, diarrhea, and premenstrual syndrome are common disorders that respond well to reflexology.

Although there is no scientific evidence that the zones and energy lines used in reflexology actually exist, reflexology may be therapeutic in that it uses touch and massage, which aid relaxation and healing.

TRANSCUTANEOUS ELECTRICAL NERVE STIMULATION (TENS)

The use of electricity to relieve pain was practiced in ancient Rome, where doctors tried to relieve gout by placing a patient's foot on an electric eel.

Today, such electrical stimulation is most widely applied through a process called transcutaneous electrical nerve stimulation, TENS, which makes use of small electrical impulses that are applied to the nerve endings just beneath the skin's surface. These seem to provide an alternative stimulus to the brain, thus blocking messages of pain. TENS is also believed to stimulate the production of endorphins, the body's own painkillers.

TENS is often recommended for sufferers of long-term or severe pain but should not be used by anyone with a pacemaker, as the electrical charge may interfere with the pacemaker's rhythm.

TENS machines are available in many doctors' offices and most physiotherapy clinics. You may also be able to purchase them from the manufacturer. Your doctor will advise you on how appropriate TENS is to your particular condition.

REFLEXOLOGY
Aches and pains throughout the body may be eased if gentle pressure is applied to the feet. A reflexology map shows which regions of the feet correspond to specific parts of the body.

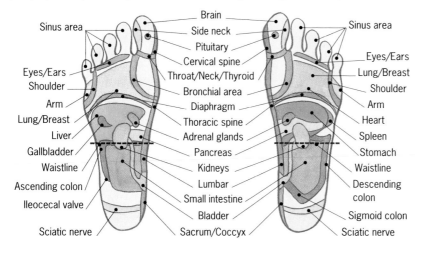

CHINESE MEDICINE

According to Chinese medicine, there are 14 invisible channels running through the body. Good health is dependent on the unimpeded flow of energy through these channels.

The emphasis in Chinese medicine is on the individual. Your symptoms will be viewed as the result of a unique set of imbalances or disharmonies within your body, and a Chinese doctor will choose specific herbs or acupuncture points to correct these and restore health.

THE THEORY

The philosophy that Chinese medicine is based upon is sometimes difficult for those brought up in the West to comprehend. One fundamental principle is that all matter in the universe, including the stars, the earth, and mankind, comes from one unified source called *tao*. Within tao there are two opposing forces: *yin*, which is seen as passive, dark, and female, and *yang*, which is seen as active, light, and male. Yin and yang exist in harmonious opposition, constantly changing and merging with each other, but always remaining in balance. This constant movement between the two creates an energy known as *chi*, or the life force.

In Chinese medicine, chi is believed to flow through the body via 14 vertical pathways, known as meridians, with each passing through a specific organ. If yin and yang become unbalanced in the body, then the flow of chi is disrupted. This can lead to blockages of energy, which Chinese doctors believe will cause ill health. An imbalance may be caused by pollution, poor nutrition, lack of exercise, an insufficient amount of rest or sleep, emotional upset, or obstructions such as tumors.

All areas of Chinese medicine are designed to restore the balance of yin and yang, thus letting chi flow smoothly and allowing the body to heal itself.

In addition to the principles of yin and yang and chi, Chinese medicine also employs the law of the five elements. The five-element theory is perhaps the hardest of all the theories to understand. Explained in simple terms, the theory states that particular organs of the body are linked with the five elements found in nature: wood, fire, earth, metal, and water, and also the seasons of the year. For example, the heart and the small intestines are associated with the summer season, which is associated with fire. When related to the natural world, disruption is seen to be caused by extreme heat, cold, wind, dampness, and dryness. By using the theories of yin and yang and the five elements, other diagnostic tools have been developed. One example of this is the concept of bodily imbalance or disharmony. If you consult a practitioner of Chinese medicine, you may be told that your symptoms are due to excess Heat, Fire, Cold, or Damp in one or more of your organs.

If these elements are viewed in relation to human illness, many similarities can be seen. An illness that is caused by Wind has symptoms that move around the body and are short lived, for example a cold. Like the wind, symptoms are mobile, almost "gusty," such as muscular spasms and dizziness.

Excess Dampness causes "heavy" symptoms, such as phlegm, while Dryness brings about chapped skin, dry, brittle hair, and dry coughs. Inflammation, skin eruptions,

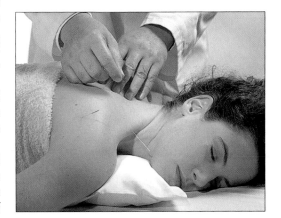

ACUPUNCTURE
To "free up" the flow of chi, fine sterile needles are inserted into the flesh and left for 10 to 30 minutes. Insertion should never be painful, but some patients report a temporary worsening of their symptoms after receiving acupuncture— practitioners say that this is a sign that the treatment is working.

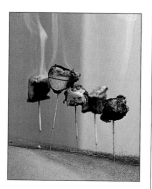

MOXIBUSTION
Common mugwort is burned on the end of acupuncture needles for a deeply penetrating effect.

and ulcers are all related to an excess of Fire, but Cold brings on pain that is "frozen" in one place and physical coldness. Just as in the natural world, where a subtle balance of the elements is vital for the maintenance of life, good health is dependent on keeping these elements in harmony.

Three basic therapies in Chinese medicine are the prescription of herbs to remedy disharmony; acupuncture, which involves the insertion of needles at specific points along the meridians in order to release the flow of chi; and acupressure, which involves applying pressure to specific points along the meridian lines.

Scientists theorize that the analgesic effects of acupuncture and acupressure may come about because the brain can receive only a certain number of messages at one time—as pressure messages reach the brain faster than pain messages, they effectively stop the pain messages from completing their journey. Modern practitioners of acupressure and acupuncture use up to 2,000 specific points.

CHINESE HERBALISM

There is a very strong tradition of using herbal remedies in China. Ancient texts have been preserved documenting the use of Chinese herbs. The *Pen Tsao*, a Chinese text written around 3000 B.C., contained some 1,000 herbal formulas, which were probably a compilation of remedies that had already been in use for thousands of years.

A Chinese herbalist does not look for any single cause or symptom in a patient but tries to find imbalances or patterns of disharmony. In order to restore the flow of chi, a special combination of herbs is prescribed, as well as dietary recommendations and sometimes acupuncture.

Certain Chinese herbs, such as Gan Cao (licorice), may be familiar to Westerners; others, such as He Shou Wu (fleece flower root), are more exotic. Chinese herbal medicine is used in the treatment of numerous conditions including migraine, cystitis, hormonal and digestive disorders, and, more recently, in the treatment of chronic skin conditions such as eczema and psoriasis.

Some herbs are toxic and may cause side effects, so consult a Chinese herbalist before taking remedies. Herbalism, however, is not a licensed specialty in North America, and some practitioners may not be well trained.

ACUPUNCTURE

It is reputed that the ancient Chinese first discovered the rudiments of acupuncture about 3,500 years ago when they observed that some warriors wounded by arrows seemed to have relief from long-standing complaints, once the wounds had healed.

As the meridians through which chi flows were identified, specific acupuncture points were mapped out. Sharp pieces of bone, bamboo, or bits of ceramic were inserted into the points to restore the flow of chi.

Although modern acupuncture is based on ancient principles, its practice is very different—acupuncturists use fine stainless steel needles that are either sterilized or disposed of after use. Insertion of the needles is quick and almost painless, although a tingling known as "needle sensation" may be felt. The practitioner may either manipulate the needles between finger and thumb, or pass an electric current through them.

Acupuncturists also practice a technique called moxibustion. This involves burning the herb mugwort to create a gentle heat close to acupuncture points. This is also believed to stimulate the flow of chi.

A first session with an acupuncturist can take up to 90 minutes, as a detailed history of the patient is built up, the tongue is examined, the arterial pulses on the wrists (three on each) are taken, and a general picture of health and demeanor is gathered.

During treatment, acupuncture needles may be left in place from 10 minutes to half an hour. If the healing effects are dramatic, only one or two sessions may be needed. Some conditions may take longer to benefit, but a degree of change should be expected after five sessions.

Asthma, depression, circulatory problems, back pain, addictions, chronic pain, and menopausal symptoms have all been treated successfully with acupuncture. Some people turn to acupuncture to help them give up

CAUTION
Some acupressure points are inappropriate if you are pregnant, frail, or elderly. Although specific instances of this are pointed out in this book, you should check with a practitioner of Chinese medicine if you are in any doubt.

smoking. Although acupuncturists should be scrupulous about using new or sterilized needles, be aware that there may be a potential danger of infection.

ACUPRESSURE

Applying pressure to acupuncture points on the body is known as acupressure and has been used for over 3,000 years to give relief from minor ailments such as headaches, stomach upsets, and insomnia. The principle of acupressure is the same as that of acupuncture, but instead of penetrating the body with needles, pressure is applied with the fingertips.

Acupressure is noninvasive and, as such, side effects are rare, although some people may experience worse symptoms before gaining relief. This is a good sign as far as practitioners are concerned, because it shows the body is trying to rebalance itself.

Applying pressure to a specific acupressure point can have effects on body organs that are a long way from that point. For instance, pressing LI 4, which is found in the web of flesh between the thumb and the forefinger, may not only help to alleviate arthritic pain in the hand, but also relieve problems in the facial area, head, and colon.

How to apply pressure

Acupressure points are found all over the body and are situated in specific places along the 14 meridian lines. The points are named according to the particular meridian they are situated on. For example, the sixth pressure point on the spleen meridian will be referred to as Sp 6. This point may be used to treat exhaustion (see page 128).

Some acupressure points are easier to locate than others. For instance, pressure point TB 17 (used to treat earache), which is found in the hollow behind the earlobes, is relatively easy to find, whereas St 36 (used to treat stomach pain), which is four finger widths below the kneecap toward the outside of the shinbone, may be more difficult to pinpoint. With practice and the aid of pressure point maps or photographs you should be able to locate points quite quickly. Alternatively, you can buy an electronic pressure point locator (see page 42). This device emits a high-pitched beep when it passes over an acupressure point—it can also be used to apply pressure.

Some acupressure points are found on both sides of the body. For instance, TB 17 can be located in the hollows behind both earlobes. If this is the case, applying pressure to points on both sides of the body will increase the therapeutic effect.

Once you have selected and located the acupressure point that is appropriate to your symptom or condition (see following chapters), use the tip of your finger or a rounded pen top to apply pressure to the point. You may find that the point feels tender. Pressure should be maintained for 20 seconds, released for 10, and then reapplied. Repeat this process up to six times.

If you are able to produce a radiating, tingling, or numb sensation from the point, it is likely that you are applying pressure to the right spot. For best results, treat most points several times over the course of a few hours. As an alternative to fingertip pressure you can use the first knuckle of your forefinger, or thumb pressure. You can even use the flat or rubber end of a pencil, but make sure that you can accurately gauge how much pressure you are applying.

MERIDIAN LINES
Chi, or life force, runs along specifically plotted channels throughout the body. It is on these pathways that acupuncture and acupressure points are located.

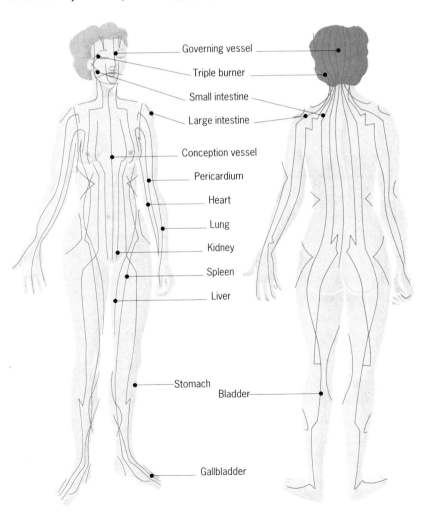

Governing vessel
Triple burner
Small intestine
Large intestine
Conception vessel
Pericardium
Heart
Lung
Kidney
Spleen
Liver
Stomach
Bladder
Gallbladder

MIND AND BODY THERAPIES

Depression and anxiety are not only debilitating problems in themselves, they also cause physical illnesses. Therapies that promote relaxation or tackle the underlying problem can help.

KNOW YOUR THERAPIST

There are many trained professionals in the counseling field, but the numerous titles may be confusing. To make sure that you are receiving the correct treatment for your problem, ask your doctor.

▶ *Psychiatrists are the only therapists who can prescribe medication; they are physicians (M.D.s) who have specialized in mental disorders.*

▶ *Clinical psychologists usually have Ph.D.s and are trained in psychological research and personality assessment. They may be qualified in a variety of therapies.*

▶ *Social workers usually have graduate degrees (M.S.W.s) and may have specific training in psychotherapy.*

▶ *Counselors, in general, tend not to have had psychological training but can offer comfort and guidance in their areas of expertise.*

The focus of many mind and body therapies is to establish the root cause of your problem and to replace your negative thoughts or low self-esteem with feelings of confidence.

COUNSELING

There is such a wide variety of different counseling techniques—everything from Gestalt therapy to transactional analysis—that it is important to consider your own goals and personal philosophy when deciding which to choose. A good therapist should have a thorough grounding in psychology, psychotherapy, or specific problem areas.

Anyone who feels unable to cope or in need of someone to talk to may benefit from counseling. The aim is to help people draw on their own resources rather than for the counselor to give direct advice. Some forms of counseling are referred to as "talking cures," which can be time consuming as clients work through their difficulties. Whether counselors work on a one-to-one basis or with groups, all aim to pinpoint and work on specific emotional problems.

Group counseling was pioneered during the First World War by William Trotter. He believed that a group provides its own dynamic force so that the counselor can interpret individual interactions within it. Group therapies now include bioenergetics, pioneered in the 1960's by an American, Dr. Alexander Lowen, in which tactile experiences such as massage are combined with talking sessions.

Counseling has proved helpful in the treatment of phobias, grief after bereavement, work-related stress, emotional problems such as depression, and, for couples, it can help resolve relationship problems.

Severe mental illnesses, such as schizophrenia, require additional medical treatment and intensive counseling.

CREATIVE VISUALIZATION

The promotion of positive thoughts may be used therapeutically to diminish negative emotions and unfounded fears and enhance self-image. Pleasure-inducing scenarios, such as a walk in the country or lying on a sunny beach, can promote relaxation. Creative visualization has been known to have suprising effects on the immune system. For instance, people with a pollen allergy may respond to the mental image of walking through a flower-filled field on a summer's day by getting hay fever.

One image that teachers of the Alexander technique (see page 45) use is that of a healthy person standing in silhouette with head and spine perfectly aligned compared with one of an ill person—stooped and round shouldered. By encouraging pupils to visualize themselves as the first rather than

A TRANQUIL LANDSCAPE
Imagining a calm, peaceful scene can slow your breathing, relax your mind, and give you a sense of general well-being.

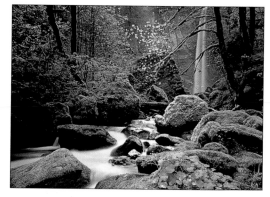

the second, the Alexander teacher fixes a positive image in their minds. Visualization may also be used to combat pain (see page 42).

Although visualization is an easily learned technique, serious or chronic pain sufferers should see a trained practitioner.

HYPNOTHERAPY

Inducing a state in which the mind becomes relaxed, focused, and receptive to suggestion is known as hypnosis. An experienced hypnotherapist can use this technique therapeutically to influence a patient's health.

Hypnotic trances were first popularized by an Austrian doctor, Franz Anton Mesmer (1734–1815), in the late 18th century (hence the word *mesmerize*). Although it was fashionable for a while, Mesmer had twice been discredited by the time of his death, and hypnotism was not widely used again until the late 1800's.

Hypnotherapy is thought to be a powerful tool in the management of stress-related disorders such as irritable bowel syndrome, anxiety, and insomnia. Research has shown that when people are hypnotized they display unique brain wave patterns that make them more receptive than normal to a hypnotist's suggestions.

At the first session, a hypnotherapist will spend time gaining the patient's trust and gathering information about the patient's life history and the problem to be tackled. The patient may be relaxed with soothing music and creative visualization. Then the hypnotherapist guides the patient into a hypnotic state where long-buried thoughts and memories can be brought to the surface of the patient's mind and explored in detail. The number of sessions needed will vary, depending on the nature of the problem.

Hypnotherapy is thought to be helpful in the treatment of migraine, skin problems, constipation, pain management, addiction, and emotional problems such as depression and eating disorders.

DID YOU KNOW?
Hypnotherapy has proved to be powerful enough to control the pain of surgery. Indeed, some doctors in the West have carried out operations such as vasectomy without the need for a conventional anesthetic.

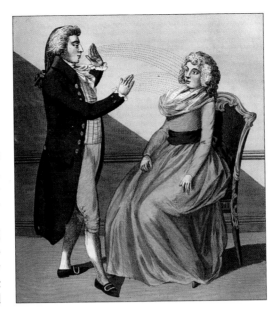

ANIMAL MAGNETISM
The 18th-century Austrian physician Franz Mesmer claimed he could perform miracle cures with what he called "animal magnetism." Although his theories were later disproved, he is credited with laying the foundation for hypnotism by demonstrating that the power of suggestion can influence health.

SEX THERAPY

Psychosexual problems are common and range from impotence, reduced sex drive, and premature ejaculation to failure to reach orgasm and vaginismus (sharp contraction of the vagina on contact).

Sexual and relationship problems are usually treated with techniques developed in the 1970's and 1980's by the sex therapists, William Masters and Virginia Johnson. Therapists first try to determine the problem through discussion—many problems that appear to have a physical origin actually stem from a lack of communication. Once communication has been reestablished, the therapist may suggest simple pleasuring techniques to practice at home. Sensual massage allows a person to gradually explore his or her physical sexuality so that repressed sexual feelings can be gently reawakened.

Sensate focusing (see page 145) allows people to receive pleasure through touch alone without the potential stress of intercourse. Both partners need to learn to express clearly what they find pleasurable before sex is attempted.

BIOFEEDBACK

By becoming aware of certain involuntary body processes, it is possible to alleviate physical symptoms caused by stress, anxiety, and a variety of ailments.

Biofeedback aims to give the patient control over his or her body. It does this with electronic devices that provide information about normally automatic body functions such as skin temperature, muscle tension, perspiration, and brain waves. These devices use sound or visual aids to report back immediately the state of the body process so that eventually the patient can consciously exert control.

For instance, electromyography (EMG) informs the patient about the muscles. Sensors attached to the skin measure electrical activity in the muscles: when the muscles are relaxed, a low hum is emitted; when they are tense, the sound is higher in pitch. Thus, when the muscles are tense, the patient can practice relaxation. Conversely, patients paralyzed by stroke may be able to improve muscular strength by learning to raise the low hum of their relaxed muscles.

Other devices used in biofeedback monitor skin temperature, which is known to drop in stressful situations, and galvanic skin response (GSR), where the level of electrical conductivity in the skin is shown on a screen. High levels of GSR are linked to the excessive sweating caused by anxiety.

Biofeedback machines are available for purchase, but it is better to start by attending sessions with a specialist. Biofeedback can be used for stress-related conditions, asthma attacks, and for reconditioning injured muscles, but should be avoided by those with endocrine disorders like diabetes.

MEDITATION

Meditation has a wide range of benefits and has been used as a path to inner peace and tranquillity for many centuries. Buddhists have been using meditation to clear their minds since the first millennium B.C. Meditation draws on our ability to induce a relaxed state by using techniques, such as deep breathing or a silent or hummed mantra (chant), which could be a single word repeated over and over.

One of the simplest forms of meditation is known as *zazen*, in which by focusing on breathing, the mind is diverted from everyday worries. The meditator sits cross-legged or in a chair with both feet flat on the floor and the back straight. This creates a physical equilibrium that makes mental focus possible. Breathing quietly through the nose, each in and out breath is counted as one. This continues until the meditator reaches a count of 10, and then the breathing cycle is repeated for about 15 minutes. Some Buddhist monks will spend up to three years on zazen before moving on to other meditation techniques. *Vispassana* meditation involves concentrating on the movement of the abdomen while breathing.

Transcendental meditation uses the tool of a mantra (the sound *om* is commonly used) to trigger the relaxation response. The technique of endlessly repeating a favorite word in order to induce a relaxed state is easy and can be done anywhere at any time—even on the bus or train on the way to work. The physical benefits of meditation include a healthier immune system because the body is less stressed. It is also used for stress-related problems such as migraine, muscular pain, asthma, and high blood pressure.

RELAXATION

Stress-related illness is a growing problem in our society—from migraine and insomnia to stomach ulcers and high blood pressure. A growing body of research shows that learning to relax can reduce the physical and psychological effects of stress on the body. There are many relaxation techniques that can be practiced easily at home (see page 114). Most of these involve learning to achieve a temporary state in which the breathing is slowed, the heart rate is lowered, and the blood flow decreased, thus allowing the body and mind to be revitalized and limiting the damaging effects of long-term stress. Research in the United States has shown that daily relaxation sessions may help break destructive habits such as alcoholism and smoking.

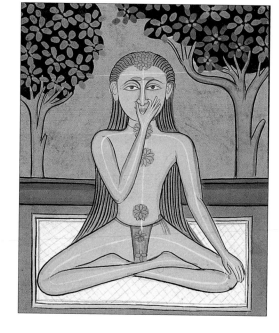

MEDITATION
This painting, from Rajasthan in northern India, shows a yogi—an adherent of yogic philosophy—practicing deep breathing and relaxation, commonly performed before entering a meditative state.

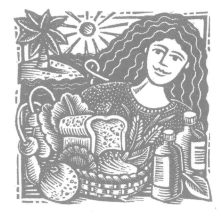

RELIEVING ACHES AND PAINS

*Massaging a strained muscle, rubbing
a bruise, taking a footbath—these are some of
the natural therapies with which we are all familiar.
They soothe the aches and pains that are part of
normal day-to-day life. For more severe or chronic
pain, natural therapies such as chiropractic or
acupuncture can give relief without the potential
side effects of some pain-relieving drugs.*

THE HEAD

Whether you are suffering from a tension headache, migraine, earache, or toothache, alternative medicine offers a wide variety of natural remedies to alleviate pain and discomfort.

CRANIOSACRAL THERAPY
The gentle manipulation of the skull bones may relieve headaches.

Headaches are usually not serious and tend to go away by themselves, but complaints such as earache or toothache may signal infection, in which case you should see a physician.

HEADACHE

The most common cause of headaches is muscular tension, brought on by stress or poor posture. Other causes include over-indulgence in food or alcohol, food intolerances, allergies, caffeine withdrawal, dental problems, eye strain, and sinus infection. Adjusting your diet or posture can help to prevent some of these headaches. Consult your doctor if you have persistent or recurrent headaches, or headaches that come and go in sudden attacks.

Relaxation
Tension headaches may be prevented or alleviated by yoga, tai chi, and the Alexander technique, therapies that relieve stress and promote physical relaxation. They also will be helpful for headaches that are caused by bad posture.

Homeopathy
Belladonna For throbbing headaches that are exacerbated by exposure to the sun or by stooping.

Ignatia For congestive, throbbing headaches, occasionally with pain extending

A cranial therapist will apply subtle pressure to the head.

to the eyes or to the sinus area, and possibly accompanied by depression.

Nux vomica For a hangover headache or a headache associated with nausea.

Acupuncture
When headaches are due to digestive problems, emotional disturbances, allergies, or muscular tension, try acupuncture.

Craniosacral therapy
Headaches may result from musculoskeletal disorders that exert pressure on nerves and blood vessels of the head. An osteopath will manipulate the muscles and spine to release tension and correct any misalignment. Craniosacral therapy is a specialized manipulation technique that treats headaches by adjusting the position of the cranial bones.

MIGRAINE
Migraine is the most severe form of headache. Symptoms include incapacitating, throbbing pain, usually on one side of the head, visual disturbances, and occasionally nausea, vomiting, or diarrhea.

A migraine is caused by the alternating constriction and dilation of veins in the head and can be triggered by factors as diverse as hormonal changes, stress, over-exertion, food intolerance, bright lights, and loud noises. An attack can last from two hours to two days, or longer.

The conventional treatment for migraine is painkillers. Herbalism, homeopathy, and reflexology are natural alternatives.

Herbalism
Feverfew is an effective herbal remedy for reducing the frequency and intensity of migraine attacks. You can either chew two fresh or freeze-dried leaves daily or take feverfew in capsule form.

Homeopathy
Spigelia For severe pain (usually on the left side of the face), pain made worse by cigarette smoke, and pain with watery eyes.

Preventing Headaches with

Naturopathy

Headaches and migraines sometimes coincide with eating a certain type of food or following a particular eating pattern. According to naturopathic principles, adjusting your diet or eating habits may bring relief.

Sensitivity to particular foods is one cause of headaches. Many people get migraines from eating cheese or chocolate, for example. If you've suffered from food-related headaches, eliminate that food from your diet for a month. If your headaches become less frequent or less severe, continue to avoid the food for another two months and then try reintroducing it gradually to see whether your tolerance to it has improved.

Naturopaths say that eating too little or eating infrequently can also cause headaches because blood sugar becomes too low or it seesaws between high and low. Headaches that occur when you miss a meal— particularly breakfast—or when you eat a lot of sugary foods, are likely due to fluctuating levels of blood sugar. If you normally skip breakfast, snack mainly on carbohydrate foods, and eat large meals later in the day, you should consider revising your eating habits so that you have a substantial breakfast and up to six small meals throughout the day. If possible, try to eliminate all sugary foods from your diet and include a high-protein food in at least two meals.

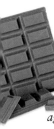

HIGH-FIBER HEADACHE RELIEF
Ease constipation-related headaches by boosting your fiber intake. Whole-grains, brown rice, oats, and wheat bran are all excellent sources of dietary fiber.

ADDING FIBER TO YOUR DIET

Some people suffer from headaches when they are constipated. To relieve discomfort, eat at least five portions of fresh fruits and vegetables every day, as well as whole-grain foods, like brown rice, whole-wheat bread and pasta, oatmeal, and wheat bran. Make any dietary changes gradually, as your intestines need time to adjust to the extra fiber.

FOODS THAT MAY CAUSE HEADACHES

Some foods contain compounds that dilate blood vessels in the head, stimulating pain-sensitive nerve endings and causing headaches. A similar effect can occur with foods to which monosodium glutamate (MSG) has been added.

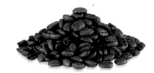

COFFEE AND TEA
Drinking, or abruptly cutting back on, caffeinated beverages is a cause of headaches.

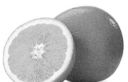

CITRUS FRUIT
Oranges, lemons, grapefruits, and limes contain a natural chemical thought to precipitate migraines.

ALCOHOL
All alcohol, but red wine in particular, is notorious for causing headaches, especially migraines.

CHOCOLATE
Caffeine and other compounds found in chocolate have been found to precipitate and aggravate headaches.

CHEESE
Cheese—especially aged cheeses, such as Brie, Camembert, and Parmesan—is high in tyramine, a naturally occurring compound that is associated with migraines.

FRUITFUL DIETS
Fresh fruits and vegetables are good sources of fiber as well as essential nutrients.

Acupressure for earache

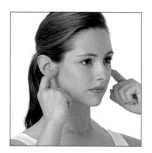

PRESSURE POINT SI 19
Press directly in front of the ear in the indentation that deepens when you open your mouth.

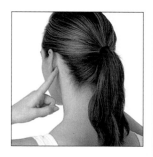

PRESSURE POINT TB 17
This is found in the hollow behind the earlobes.

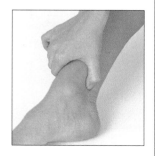

PRESSURE POINT KID 3
This point is one finger width above the hollow between the inside of the ankle bone and the Achilles tendon.

Sanguinaria For pain that spreads from the base of the skull to the right eye and is accompanied by hot flashes.
Kali bichromicum For migraine preceded by visual disturbances.

Reflexology
Sensitive spots on your feet may point to the underlying cause of your migraine. A problem in the colon, for example, may cause headache; a reflexologist will treat the problem by massaging the area of your foot that corresponds to the colon.

EARACHE
Pain in the ear may result from the buildup of earwax, a disorder affecting an area near the ear, or it may be due to a bacterial infection. An acute infection of the inner ear, if left untreated, can result in perforation of the eardrum and hearing loss. Always consult a doctor before treating an earache with natural remedies.

Conventional treatment to remove excess wax consists of syringing and, for an infection, antibiotics. Do not remove wax by poking objects into the ear. Natural therapies include hydrotherapy, acupressure, and herbalism for pain relief, and naturopathy and craniosacral therapy to solve any underlying problem.

Hydrotherapy
For immediate relief, hold a hot compress against the ear. The compress should be as hot as is comfortable and left against the ear until it cools. This will stimulate the circulation of blood to the area and help to alleviate the pain.

Acupressure
For relief from earache that is due to exposure to cold or to changes in water or air pressure, try applying pressure to SI 19, TB 17, or Kid 3. In each case, apply pressure for 30 seconds with slight finger vibration. Repeat six times at 20-second intervals.

Herbalism
Put two drops of mullein flower oil on a piece of cotton and gently insert it into the affected ear. Make sure that you do not force it too far into the ear canal.

Echinacea has mild anti-inflammatory qualities and is recommended for treating ear infections; goldenrod and goldenseal ease earache. All are available in dried, tincture, or tablet form. Do not take goldenseal if you are pregnant or if you are suffering from hypertension.

Naturopathy
For repeated infections, naturopaths recommend zinc and vitamins B, C, and E. Foods rich in these nutrients include dairy products, green vegetables, whole-grain breads, citrus fruits, and seafood.

Craniosacral therapy
Pain in the ear that has started after an injury to the head or the spine may be particularly responsive to gentle manipulation of the bones in the skull.

TOOTHACHE
Pain in the teeth and gums is usually caused by decay, infection, or inflammation and should be treated by a dentist as quickly as possible. For temporary pain relief, or for discomfort or soreness after you have received dental care, acupressure, herbalism, or homeopathy can help.

Acupressure
Deep pressure should be applied to LI 4, known as the great eliminator (see page 68), the point at the center of the webbing between your thumb and index finger. Do not use this point during pregnancy.

Herbalism
Apply tincture of myrrh or oil of cloves to the gum around the aching tooth (avoid myrrh during pregnancy). For a cavity, a small plug of cotton soaked in oil of cloves can help. Clove oil, well recognized for its anesthetic properties, contains eugenol, a volatile oil that dentists use to numb pain.

Homeopathy
Mercurius solubilis For pain that abates at night, returns in the morning, and is made worse by hot or cold drinks.
Arnica For bleeding and discomfort after dental treatment and for pain in the right upper jaw, extending to the ear.
Aconite For pain on the left side of the jaw, made worse by cold and accompanied by red cheeks, and the shock of dental surgery.

> **CAUTION**
> *Throbbing pain accompanied by swelling around the gum and tenderness of the tooth, sometimes complicated by a swollen face and neck and a high temperature, may be symptoms of a tooth abscess and require emergency treatment by a dentist.*

THE JOINTS, MUSCLES, AND TENDONS

Incorrect posture, injuries, or disease can cause painful joints, muscles, and tendons. Instead of relying on painkillers, many people prefer natural therapies for safe and effective relief.

Generally speaking, painful joints and muscles can be eased through a combination of massage—coupled with essential oils—and any one of many different forms of gentle exercise; yoga and tai chi may be especially efficacious.

JOINT PAIN
Pain in the knees, wrists, elbows, hips, and other joints can arise from osteoarthritis, rheumatoid arthritis, and sprains due to accidents or incorrect exercising, for example. If you suffer from persistently painful joints, consult your doctor.

Conventional treatment for joint pain includes painkilling or anti-inflammatory drugs, physiotherapy, and, occasionally, surgery. To relieve discomfort, try homeopathy, regular exercise, Chinese medicine, or hydrotherapy.

Homeopathy
Rhus toxicodendron For joint pain that becomes worse with resting, improves with sustained movement, is exacerbated by cold and damp conditions, and becomes better in a warm environment.

Nux vomica For joint pain that is accompanied by irritability; symptoms are at their worst in the early morning and in the cold but get better in the evening and in warm temperatures.

Bryonia For stiff, swollen joints that are more painful after movement and exposure to heat and less painful after resting and exposure to cold.

Exercise
Regular gentle exercise, such as swimming, is one of the best ways to keep your joints healthy and flexible. Even simple ankle and wrist circling while you are sitting can be helpful. If you suffer from arthritis (see page 104), a physiotherapist is a good person to consult for an exercise program.

Chinese medicine
Since no two people have exactly the same symptoms, a practitioner of Chinese medicine will tailor an individual course of treatment. Both herbs and acupuncture may be prescribed to relieve pain.

Hydrotherapy
Applying hot and cold compresses can help increase circulation: use ice packs for joint pain that is hot or burning, hot towels for pain that is alleviated by warmth, and hot towels and ice packs alternately for general stiffness in your joints.

CARPAL TUNNEL SYNDROME
The pain, tingling, or numbness of the fingers that can result from a repeated wrist movement, such as typing, playing a violin, or hitting a tennis ball, is commonly known as carpal tunnel syndrome or repetitive stress injury (RSI). Symptoms are caused by pressure on the median nerve of the wrist, leading to inflammation and discomfort that may progress to shooting pain in the forearm and shoulder.

Conventional treatment includes rest, wrist splints, and occupational therapy. A doctor may prescribe painkillers, anti-inflammatory drugs, or diuretics, and may occasionally recommend surgery. Try natural therapies such as acupressure, exercise, naturopathy, hydrotherapy, and homeopathy for relief.

Acupressure
Three points are recommended to relieve carpal tunnel syndrome: P 6 (see page 133), SI 3, and LI 11. P 6 is on the middle of the inside of the forearm, two to three finger widths up from the wrist crease. Applying

Acupressure for RSI

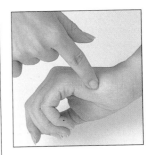

PRESSURE POINT SI 3
This can be found by running a finger down from the base of the little finger until you feel a notch in the bone roughly halfway between the knuckle and the wrist crease. Apply steady pressure.

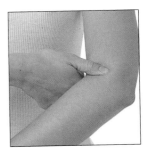

PRESSURE POINT LI 11
Bend the arm at a right angle. Locate the highest point on the elbow crease and apply pressure.

Acupressure for muscle pain

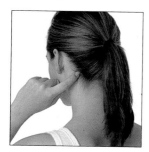

PRESSURE POINT GB 20
This is at the base of the skull on either side of the top of the spine in the hollows between the two large neck muscles. Tilt your head back against your finger.

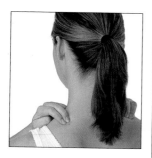

PRESSURE POINT GB 21
This is halfway between the base of the neck and the edge of shoulder, slightly to the back. Avoid using GB 21 if you are pregnant.

pressure to P 6 and SI 3 should help alleviate wrist pain; press LI 11 for elbow pain.

Exercise
Regular hand and wrist exercises can relieve the numbness and tingling of carpal tunnel syndrome. Start by clenching your fists and then spreading your fingers out. Repeat this 20 times. Next, make circles with your hands, rotating around the wrist. Do this for about two minutes. Finally, repeat both exercises with your hands above your head. Practice this sequence of movements several times each day.

Naturopathy
If you are suffering from a buildup of fluid around the wrist, vitamin B_6 may help to reduce swelling. Try to eat foods that are rich in vitamin B_6 such as meat, fish, poultry, and bananas, or take a vitamin B_6 supplement.

Hydrotherapy
Alternating hot and cold compresses to the wrist will stimulate circulation: apply a towel dipped in hot water for three to four minutes. Follow this with a cold compress for about 40 seconds. Repeat this process five to six times as often as necessary to relieve discomfort.

Homeopathy
Causticum For pain that is relieved by heat and rubbing, and associated with tingling or numbness.

MUSCLE PAIN
Torn or strained muscles caused by overexertion or accident commonly result in mild discomfort to disabling agony. Such injuries often take several weeks to heal and can leave muscles weakened. Conventional treatments include painkilling drugs, muscle relaxants, anti-inflammatory drugs, physiotherapy, and electrical stimulation. Natural therapies are aromatherapy massage, acupressure, homeopathy, acupuncture, and naturopathy.

Aromatherapy
Massaging the affected muscle with essential oils can be very soothing. Add 4 drops of marjoram oil, 6 drops of eucalyptus oil, and 5 drops of rosemary oil to 1½ fluid ounces (3 tablespoons) of a base oil. Warm the oil in your hands before applying it to the skin. If a painful muscle is inaccessible ask someone to massage it for you. Make sure you are comfortable before you begin a massage.

Soaking the entire body in an aromatherapy bath can also help ease discomfort. Add two drops each of rosemary, eucalyptus, and lavender oils to warm water.

Acupressure
Apply steady pressure to points GB 20 and 21, and Bl 2 (see page 46). Bl 2 is at the ends of the eyebrows on either side of the nose. Avoid using GB 21 during pregnancy.

Homeopathy
Arnica For painful, overworked muscles after strenuous exercise.

Acupuncture
Muscle pain may be helped by acupuncture in two ways: practitioners of Chinese medicine believe that it increases the flow of vital Energy to the affected area and encourages healing; and, according to some scientists, it increases the level of endorphins (the body's natural painkillers) in the bloodstream.

Naturopathy
Chronic muscle soreness and fatigue may result from a deficiency of vitamins B, C, and E and may also be a symptom of iron deficiency anemia. Make sure that your diet contains plenty of whole-grain cereals, citrus fruits, and leafy green vegetables. Alternatively, take a vitamin and mineral supplement, but remember that supplements do not contain all the nutrients that a healthy diet provides. Consult a doctor before taking vitamin E if you have heart disease or hypertension.

CRAMP
When muscle fibers contract and go into spasm, a painful cramp occurs. Cramps can result from the buildup of lactic acid in muscles that are overexerted or chronically tense. Other causes include insufficient dietary minerals and repetitive actions, such as writing. Leg cramps at night are common. Massage and homeopathy can be used for immediate pain relief; a healthy diet and regular exercise may provide more permanent freedom from pain.

Massage
The cramped muscle should be stretched as far as possible against the spasm and massaged vigorously using both effleurage and petrissage (see opposite page). This action increases the blood supply to the muscles and disperses any buildup of lactic acid.

Homeopathy
Cuprum met For cramp that affects the fingers, legs, and toes.

Easing Stiff Muscles with

Massage Techniques

Kneading, pounding, and manipulating the muscles, tendons, and ligaments releases tension and improves circulation. Increased blood flow brings oxygen to tissues and helps disperse toxins, thus relieving pain and promoting healing.

When muscles are overworked or tensed, whether from poor posture, overstraining, or as a response to stress, chronic muscle pain can develop. Sore muscles can be massaged with a few basic techniques that are not hard to learn. If the muscles are very painful, begin gently and gradually progress to deeper strokes.

GIVING A MASSAGE

▶ *Make sure the person being massaged is warm and relaxed.*
▶ *Use the weight of your body to press down—not just your arms.*
▶ *Vary the speed and type of massage strokes.*
▶ *Use enough oil to let your hands glide over the skin.*

MASSAGING AWAY MUSCLE PAIN

The most widely used massage stroke is effleurage. This is a smooth, flowing stroke designed to relax the person being massaged. Effleurage is useful for linking together other more intensive massage strokes, including petrissage, percussion, and friction.

Although massage is usually a safe therapy, it should be avoided if you have varicose veins, any sort of skin problem, including cuts and burns, or a serious disease such as cancer or osteoporosis.

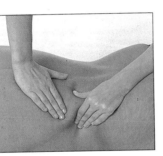

PETRISSAGE
Sometimes called kneading, wringing, or rolling, this squeezing movement is applied across the muscle fibers. It helps break up knots and tension spots.

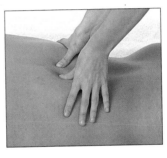

FRICTION
For the friction stroke, a variation of petrissage, the thumbs and fingers are used to apply small circular movements either in a single spot or in a series of spots.

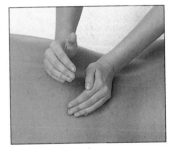

PERCUSSION
Striking with the sides of the hands, percussion, which is also known as tapotement or hacking, can be stimulating (lasting under two minutes) or relaxing (over two minutes).

EFFLEURAGE
Use both hands to apply long, gliding strokes that follow the direction of the muscle fibers. Strokes should always be toward the heart.

Naturopathy

Calcium is essential for the action of muscle fibers, and a deficiency may lead to muscle cramps. Dairy products are a good source of calcium, particularly low-fat milk and cheese; calcium can also be obtained from dark green leafy vegetables, canned sardines and salmon with bones, and dried beans. Effective calcium absorption depends on the presence of other vitamins and minerals, particularly vitamin D, and a balanced diet can ensure that they are present. Potassium is another mineral that is important for muscle function—good sources include whole-grain cereals and breads, potatoes, bananas, oranges, prunes, and dried apricots. Magnesium—found in nuts, milk, fish, legumes, and green vegetables—may also help prevent muscle cramps.

Exercise

Sedentary people are more prone to muscle cramps. Moderate exercise like walking, swimming, or yoga will keep muscles toned and less likely to cramp.

STIFF NECK

Neck pain can be caused by injury, bad posture, arthritis, sleeping or working in an awkward position, and inadvertent tensing of muscles due to stress and anxiety. Waste products, such as lactic acid, may build up in tense, overworked muscles and, if they are not removed by the blood, can cause pain and stiffness.

Aromatherapy should help relieve discomfort and the Alexander technique can correct your posture and prevent pain and stiffness.

Aromatherapy

Add lavender or eucalyptus essential oil to a base massage oil (see page 21) and apply to the skin using firm, stroking movements along the back and sides of the neck and the tops of the shoulders. Use small fingertip circles of pressure to get rid of tight knots.

Alexander technique

Chronic stiffness and pain as a result of bad posture may be eased with the help of a certified practitioner, who will use simple exercises to correct the way you sit, stand, and walk (see page 45).

> ## WARNING
>
> *Occasionally, a stiff neck may be accompanied by a fever, headache, and nausea, which can indicate a serious condition such as meningitis. If you develop these symptoms, consult your doctor without delay.*

YOGA MOVEMENTS FOR A STIFF NECK

The muscles of the neck and shoulders are especially prone to becoming tense and stiff. There are many yoga poses, such as the plow, the cobra, and the lion, that promote relaxation of these muscles. The movements below are gentle and will help to increase the flexibility of your neck if practiced daily.

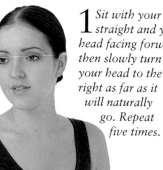
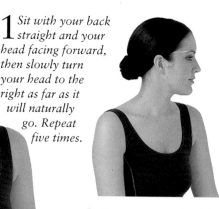

1 *Sit with your back straight and your head facing forward, then slowly turn your head to the right as far as it will naturally go. Repeat five times.*

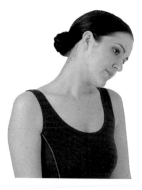

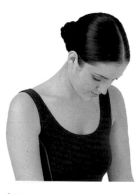

2 *Now turn your head five times to the left. Each time you turn your head, you should find that it goes a little farther.*

3 *Next, let your head drop toward one shoulder, then the other. Do not force it— just let your muscles relax. Repeat five times.*

4 *Let your head drop gently forward toward your chest. Feel the muscles at the back of your neck relax for a count of five.*

BACKACHE

Pain anywhere along the spine from the base of the skull to the tailbone constitutes backache. The pain can be acute or chronic and have numerous causes, many of which are not fully understood. Backache may result from muscle strain or it may be due to more serious problems like a slipped disk, osteoarthritis, or osteoporosis. Sometimes backache is caused by stress-related muscle tension or a viral infection such as flu. Although in many cases the pain will disappear with bed rest, your doctor may prescribe an analgesic or muscle relaxant. Physiotherapy can also help. Many natural therapies ease or prevent back pain.

Acupressure
For lower backache, especially if the pain radiates down the leg, try firm pressure on Bl 47 or Bl 23. Maintain the pressure for about 30 seconds—slight vibration of the finger will increase the sensation—then release and repeat after 20 seconds.

Massage
If back pain is muscular in origin, a massage from a professional therapist or even a friend can ease pain and discomfort (see page 39).

Rolfing is a form of very deep massage using the fingers, knuckles, and elbows, which practitioners say eases complaints that haven't responded to other therapies, especially where stress and emotional problems are also involved. Rolfing should be performed only by a qualified practitioner.

Tai chi and yoga
Toned muscles, good posture, and general fitness will help prevent backache. Tai chi and yoga are both excellent therapies for sufferers of chronic back pain because, in addition to improving flexibility and fitness, they relieve pain by relaxing muscles and reducing stress. Some experts suggest that as many as 98 percent of back pain sufferers could benefit from practicing yoga regularly. A few basic yoga poses (see page 43) performed each day should keep your back strong and pain-free.

If you are in severe pain, consult your doctor before attempting any physical exercise.

Alexander technique
A method of reeducating the body, the Alexander technique (see page 45) involves adjusting body posture to relieve chronic back pain and muscle tension, and increase range of motion. To learn the technique properly, go to a certified instructor, who will teach you how to relax your muscles and adjust your posture when sitting, standing, and moving by using simple exercises, touch, and verbal instruction.

Exercise
Increase bone strength with regular weight-bearing exercise, which will reduce the risk for diseases such as osteoporosis (see page 108). Low-impact aerobics, dancing, or walking three times a week is ideal. Yoga, stretches, and sit-ups will strengthen lower back muscles so they can support your spine adequately. In addition, exercise will promote the release of endorphins (these are natural substances in the body that act as painkillers) into the bloodstream. A physiotherapist can design an exercise program specifically to prevent back pain.

Chinese medicine
Backache may arise from a blockage or shortage of Energy caused by either a constitutional weakness or strained muscles. A shortage of Energy is particularly amenable to treatment with Chinese herbs and acupuncture. Consult a practitioner of Chinese medicine for advice.

Osteopathy
The manipulation of the spine by a trained practitioner to correct the alignment of the spinal vertebrae is a popular and effective way of treating many types of back pain.

A treatment session might begin with massage or transcutaneous electrical nerve stimulation (TENS) to relax the muscles and reduce pain before manipulation. The osteopath will then try to reeducate the ligaments and muscles, and correct the alignment of bones by gently levering one part of the body against another.

Bear in mind that manipulative therapies such as osteopathy and chiropractic are dangerous if you have low bone mass or osteoporosis (see page 108). Osteoporosis is a disease in which bone density declines to a point where bones become brittle and fracture easily.

continued on page 44

Acupressure for backache

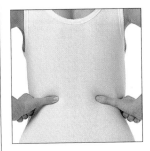

PRESSURE POINT BL 47
This point is found on the lower back (between the second and third lumbar vertebrae), four finger widths away from the spine at waist level.

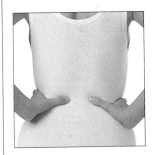

PRESSURE POINT BL 23
This is also found on the lower back, but it is two finger widths nearer to the spine than point Bl 47 (see above).

Natural Pain Relief

Natural therapies aim to encourage the body's innate healing powers, but many can also be used to alleviate pain. Most techniques are easy to learn and practice at home, and none will cause the side effects common to many painkilling drugs.

ZONE THERAPY

Massaging points on the hands may help relieve pain in the same way that pressing points on the body does in acupressure. Using the thumb of one hand, massage the inner edge of the other palm, just below the fingers. Work toward the outer edge of the hand, massaging each joint in turn. Having completed one "panel" of the palm, go down to the next. Repeat on any sensitive points.

ACUPRESSURE

You can locate and stimulate specific acupressure points by using a hand-held, battery-operated device known as an electronic pressure point finder. The device emits a low-powered electronic pulse when it passes over the correct spot and may be useful in relieving many types of pain.

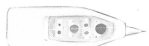

ELECTRONIC PRESSURE POINT FINDER
Once this device locates a point, hold it in place for 20 seconds or more.

PRESSURE POINT MAP
"Maps" of the body's pressure points are sold in specialist shops. This diagram gives an indication of some of the points on the front of the body, particularly those useful for pain relief.

Endorphins are naturally occurring substances in the body that block pain signals relayed to the brain. These "feel good" chemicals are released when the nerve cells are stimulated and during exercise. Acupuncture and acupressure may also activate their release. These therapies, together with zone therapy, which treats pain occurring elsewhere in the body by palm massage, may greatly reduce the need for conventional painkilling drugs, like aspirin or ibuprofen. Many people have found that relaxation and creative visualization techniques have enabled them to use their minds alone to control levels of pain.

THE POWER OF THE MIND

For individuals who suffer from chronic pain due to arthritis or neuralgia, for example, creative visualization may be helpful. To practice this technique, you need to be relaxed—if you react to pain by tensing your body, you may exacerbate your symptoms.

Make sure you are warm and comfortable, and start by practicing the breathing exercises on page 114. Close your eyes and concentrate on the area of your body where the pain is centered.

As you breathe, imagine the breath going in and out of the painful area. As you inhale, imagine a warm glow healing the pain, and as you exhale, imagine the pain being expelled. Some people imagine their pain as an object with a specific color, size, and texture. If you can do this, manipulate the pain mentally: alter its color, shape, and size in your mind, and then try to make it smaller.

If pain is caused by infection, imagine a battle between your healthy immune cells and the bacteria or virus. Above all, have confidence in your natural ability to control pain and fight disease.

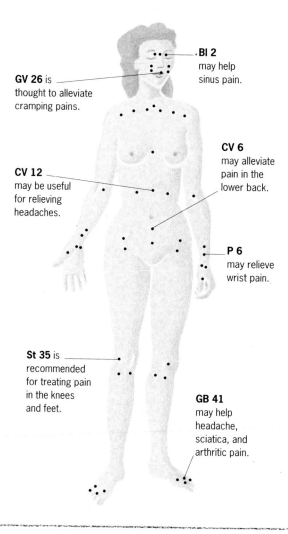

GV 26 is thought to alleviate cramping pains.

BI 2 may help sinus pain.

CV 6 may alleviate pain in the lower back.

CV 12 is may be useful for relieving headaches.

P 6 may relieve wrist pain.

St 35 is recommended for treating pain in the knees and feet.

GB 41 may help headache, sciatica, and arthritic pain.

RELIEVING PAIN WITH YOGA

Yoga is a gentle form of exercise that can help prevent pain by improving posture and increasing overall flexibility. It can ease existing pain by gently stretching sore muscles. This sequence of yoga poses, called Sun Salutation, is good for alleviating mild muscular aches and pains.

Each pose should be done in time with your breathing. After completing these seven poses, exhale and return to position five; inhale and return to position four; exhale and return to position three; then inhale and return to position two. Finally, exhale and return to the original praying position. Try to practice Sun Salutation at least once a day, preferably first thing in the morning.

3 *Exhale, lean forward and try to touch the ground (do not force it) with the palms of your hands. Relax the muscles in your neck.*

1 *Stand up straight and relaxed with your feet together and your hands in a prayer position.*

2 *Inhale deeply and raise your arms above your head.*

4 *Inhale, bend your left knee forward, and stretch your right leg backward. Keep your palms flat on the floor and your arms straight.*

5 *Move your left foot back to meet your right foot, and raise your body into an arch. Exhale.*

6 *Lower your body slowly to the floor, leading with your knees and shoulders.*

7 *Inhale and lift your chest and shoulders up, keeping your abdomen on the floor.*

43

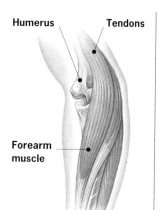

Humerus **Tendons**

Forearm muscle

THE TENDONS
Fibrous cords that join muscle to bone or muscle to muscle, tendons are strong and flexible, but inelastic.

LOOKING AFTER YOUR BACK

Obesity can cause or exacerbate back pain, so keep your weight down, or, if you are overweight, consult your doctor about a diet and exercise program. At all times make sure that you are standing and sitting correctly. When you stand, your head should be in line with your torso and the balls of your feet. When sitting, a chair should support the whole of your spine.

Use a mattress that's firm and supportive rather than sagging and soft, and a pillow that keeps your head, neck, and back in alignment.

When you bend to pick things up, bend at the knees, keeping your spine straight. As you lift an object, keep it close to your body, especially if it is heavy. Take the weight on your legs so that you don't strain your back.

Plan your work so that you don't sit or stand in one position for too long. If this is not possible, take regular breaks and gently stretch your muscles.

Chiropractic

If you consult a chiropractor about pain, the initial diagnosis will involve X-rays of the spine. Having established the cause of your backache, a chiropractor will manipulate your spine using short, sharp, thrusting movements.

MANIPULATION
You may receive treatment on a specially designed chiropractic couch. Some manipulations are carried out while you are lying down, others while you are standing or sitting.

The sudden thrusting movements used in chiropractic will pull and relax muscles that are in spasm.

TENDINITIS

Inflammation of the tendons (the tissue that joins muscle to bone or muscle to muscle) is known as tendinitis, which occurs when a tendon is injured or overused. It is common when you overdo an activity that constantly repeats the same movements, or have incorrect posture while lifting or exercising.

The tendons that are most commonly affected by tendinitis are those located in the shoulder, heel, knee, and elbow. Symptoms include swelling, tenderness, pain, and restricted movement.

Inflamed tendons on the outside of the elbow are referred to as tennis elbow, since they can result from the repetitive movements involved in playing tennis.

Conventional treatment usually consists of rest, anti-inflammatory drugs, and, sometimes, cortisone injections. Herbalism, gentle massage, and naturopathic remedies may also be helpful.

Herbalism

Arnica is a useful herb for tendinitis. Apply arnica cream to the affected area, or soak a pad in dilute tincture and use as a compress. Do not take arnica internally. Apply witch hazel water or solution after any swelling has gone down.

Hot and cold compresses of turmeric (see page 17) may also help reduce inflammation by increasing blood circulation. Hot compresses are good for chronic cases of tendinitis, while cold compresses are good for acute cases. (Compresses will help even without the addition of turmeric.) Curcumin, a compound extracted from the turmeric root, is available in tablets of turmeric root extract, standardized for their curcumin contents.

Massage

After resting the injured part of the body for a few days, try a gentle massage. If the arm is affected, start with light effleurage on the whole arm followed by petrissage strokes on the elbow area (see page 39). Use deep thumb pressure only as the injury begins to heal and the pain abates. Professional massage may be helpful.

Naturopathy

Eat foods that are rich in vitamin C, vitamin E, beta carotene, and zinc because they are believed to heal damaged tissue. Leafy green vegetables, citrus fruits, whole-grain cereals, liver, dairy products, and lentils are good sources of these nutrients.

The Alexander Technique

Widely advocated as a means of preventing backache, the Alexander technique is a method of mental and physical reeducation that improves posture and teaches you how to use your body to its best advantage.

According to teachers of the Alexander technique, many people have bad sitting postures that develop over time, with the damage beginning in childhood. Most young children have good posture and their bodies are naturally aligned. When they go to school, however, they acquire bad habits. When children sit at a desk they tend to adopt a slumped posture with the head bent forward, looking down. This position becomes ingrained and when a child looks up, the head is raised but the collapsed position remains, increasing overall body shortening. Such bad habits lead the muscles in the back and neck to contract and cause tension, fatigue, pain, and stiffness.

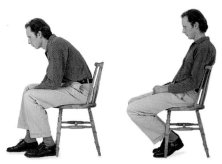

POOR POSTURE
Backache is likely if you spend a lot of time sitting incorrectly. Both of these postures put unnecessary stress on the spine, neck, and shoulders because the head is tipped forward and the feet do not give adequate support to the body.

HOW TO IMPROVE YOUR SITTING POSTURE

Good sitting posture can reduce muscle tension in the body and restore the vertebrae to their correct alignment. Instead of being compressed, the abdomen will be open and the chest will be "widened," enabling you to breathe freely and relax more completely.

Observe the way your body is arranged when you are sitting. Is your torso slumped? Is your back bent and are your shoulder muscles tense? Is your head on one side or being supported by your hand? Are your legs crossed? Does your body feel stiff? Try putting your hands on your abdomen—is it compressed? If you answer yes to all or even some of these questions, awareness of these bad habits will help you overcome them.

Rather than physically forcing your shoulders to drop, your head to rise, and your spine to straighten, simply concentrate on not holding on to a bent neck and hunched shoulders.

SITTING CORRECTLY
Imagine your head rising, your shoulders relaxing, and your spine lengthening. Let your body naturally adopt the correct position.

Feel your neck and spine become free and your head rise up.

Completely relax your shoulders. Don't try to force them back or down.

Place your hands loosely on your thighs with your palms upturned.

Your knees should be kept apart and at a 90° angle. Your calves should be perpendicular to the floor.

Take the weight of your torso on the two bones at the bottom of your pelvis, known as the sit bones. Make sure that the weight is evenly distributed between them.

Rest the soles of your feet flat on the floor.

THE NERVES

The pain of neuralgia can be debilitating. Many who suffer from nerve pain can benefit from natural remedies that use the power of the mind and body to control discomfort.

Acupressure for neuralgia

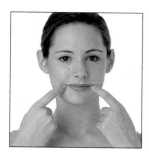

PRESSURE POINT ST 4
Press the points at the corners of the mouth with your index fingers.

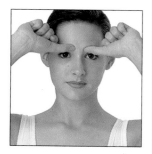

PRESSURE POINT BL 2
Place your thumbs at the edge of each eyebrow on either side of your nose. Apply steady pressure by leaning your head against your thumbs.

Nerve pain may be difficult to treat, and some sufferers find that even surgery fails to help relieve pain. Acupressure may help facial neuralgia; hydrotherapy and homeopathy can be practiced at home.

NEURALGIA

Nerve pain or neuralgia is caused by irritation or injury and can affect any nerve in the body. It is often a chronic problem, experienced as brief attacks of pain or numb, tingling, or burning sensations. A type of neuralgia known as postherpetic neuralgia can occur after a bout of shingles. Neuralgia typically affects the face, the back of the tongue, the middle ear, or the backs of the legs.

Doctors recommend pain relief medications such as aspirin or acetaminophen. Occasionally, surgery may be recommended. Of the natural remedies, acupressure, hydrotherapy, aromatherapy, and meditation may help.

Acupressure
Try applying steady pressure to points St 4 or Bl 2. This may help relieve the pain of facial neuralgia.

Hydrotherapy
Hot or cold compresses (see page 17) may provide temporary pain relief, unless you find that extremes of temperature trigger or exacerbate neuralgia attacks.

Aromatherapy
Nervine essences—those that calm the nervous system—can be used in inhalations or baths, or they can be mixed with a bland carrier oil (sweet almond or soybean) to make massage oils. Try basil, clove, eucalyptus, or lavender essential oils.

Meditation
Sometimes there is no alternative other than learning to live with chronic pain. A therapy known as mindfulness meditation has helped many people cope. It involves sitting quietly for 45 minutes once or twice every day, and monitoring your pain. Gradually, you learn to recognize that the intensity of pain is not constant, but occurs in peaks and troughs. This awareness can give you a greater sense of control over pain and increase your resilience and enthusiasm for day-to-day activities.

SCIATICA

The sciatic nerve is the longest, thickest nerve in your body. It emerges from several spinal nerves, passes under the muscle in the buttocks, and extends down each leg. Pain—especially shooting pain—numbness, or tingling anywhere along the nerve pathway is called sciatica and is a type of neuralgia. The usual cause is pressure from a vertebra on one of the spinal nerves that form the sciatic nerve. The pain may be worse at night, on sudden movement, or after sitting down. Medical treatments include painkillers, bed rest, and moist heat. In severe cases, when walking becomes difficult, surgery may be an option. Natural remedies such as hydrotherapy and homeopathy are recommended to alleviate pain.

Hydrotherapy
Alternate applications of hot and cold compresses may be helpful. The applications should be of equal duration and last no longer than 10 minutes.

Homeopathy
Lycopodium For right-sided symptoms that come and go suddenly, have a gradual onset, and include numbness or tingling.
Kali bichromicum For shooting pain, left-sided pain, and pain that is worse in the morning and relieved by moving around.
Rhus toxicodendron For pain that is relieved by warmth and movement.
Hypericum For excessive, spasmodic pain triggered by injury or trauma.

CHAPTER 3

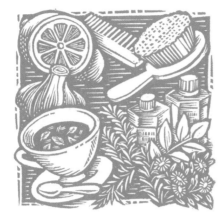

SKIN, HAIR, AND NAIL PROBLEMS

Some of our earliest medical preparations were ointments, lotions, and balms for the care of the skin and the hair. Today, the topical application of herbs and diluted essential oils to the skin is thought to relieve complaints as diverse as cold sores and athlete's foot. Therapies such as naturopathy can improve the health of the skin, hair, and nails by correcting the diet.

THE SKIN

Soothing herbs can be especially helpful in treating skin complaints. Western herbalists and practitioners of Chinese medicine recommend an array of time-tested herbal remedies.

Rehydrating face packs
If you suffer from dry skin, make a face pack using honey and either a mashed avocado or raw egg yolk. Avoid the eye area when applying. Leave on the face for approximately 10 to 15 minutes. Repeat once a week.

Some skin problems, such as warts, are relatively painless but need to be treated because they are unsightly or annoying; others, such as boils and abscesses, cause serious discomfort and demand immediate attention.

ITCHY SKIN

Irritated, prickly, or itchy skin is called pruritus. It is a common symptom of infections like chickenpox; skin ailments, such as eczema; and allergic reactions to chemicals, metals, clothing, or foods. Itchiness may also indicate more serious illnesses, like hepatitis or diabetes, or it may be a symptom of stress.

Conventional treatments for pruritus include emollients (lotions or creams), cooling preparations such as calamine lotion, or local anesthetics that block nerve signals to the brain. For itchiness due to an allergy, antihistamines or steroids are often prescribed. Herbalism, hydrotherapy, and Chinese herbalism may relieve discomfort.

Herbalism
For pruritus due to eczema, an herbalist may prescribe red clover. Self-help remedies for dry, itchy skin include calendula cream with chamomile, lavender, or peppermint essential oil added (two to three drops to 1 teaspoon of cream), or chickweed cream—simply rub into the affected area. Both calendula and chickweed creams are available from health food stores. Fresh *Aloe vera* gel squeezed from a leaf and comfrey compresses also relieve itching. (Do not take comfrey internally.)

Hydrotherapy
You can alleviate itchiness by applying compresses made with cold water to the affected skin. You can also try soaking for 20 to 30 minutes in warm water (just above room temperature). Add either 1 cup sodium bicarbonate (baking soda), or 1 cup each of finely ground oatmeal and cornstarch to your bathwater.

Chinese herbalism
Itchy skin is regarded by practitioners of Chinese medicine as a sign of Heat and Wind in the body (see page 27). They recommend herbs to expel Wind and cool the Blood. Such remedies include Jin Yin Hua (honeysuckle flowers), Lian Qiao (forsythia fruit), Bo He (peppermint), and Chan Tui (cicada shells). If dry or itchy skin is due to a deficiency in the Blood, then Blood-nourishing herbs are prescribed. These might include Sheng Di Huang (Chinese foxglove root, also known as raw rehmannia), Dang Gui (Chinese angelica root), and Bai Shao Yao (white peony root).

DRY, CHAPPED, OR SORE SKIN

Some people have naturally dry skin or skin that chaps easily in the cold. But dry, irritated, or inflamed skin that itches may also be a sign of an underlying condition such as dermatitis or eczema. Allergic reactions, stress, dry climates, hot and cold temperatures, woollen clothing, and environmental pollutants can cause both conditions.

The main treatment for dryness and irritation is an emollient cream or lotion that

COOLING COMPRESS FOR ITCHY SKIN

Cucumber juice cools the skin and alleviates itchiness. Apply to the affected area as a compress or lotion. The cucumber peel can also be applied to the skin.

EXTRACTING THE JUICE
Peel and slice a cucumber, leave it in a bowl for two hours, and then press the slices through cheesecloth.

soothes and rehydrates your skin. For more serious conditions, your doctor may prescribe a steroid cream, which will relieve itchiness and inflammation, but long-term use is inadvisable. Natural therapies for dry, chapped, or irritated skin include herbalism and naturopathy.

Herbalism

Calendula, chickweed, chamomile, *Aloe vera*, marsh mallow, and evening primrose can be applied externally to relieve dry or irritated skin. These herbs may be bought as creams, or you can make your own cream or ointment (see page 17). Calendula and St. John's wort cream are also soothing. Apply a wet chamomile tea bag to the affected area to ease irritation or fresh *Aloe vera* gel if skin is weeping. Herbalists also recommend infusions or decoctions of herbs such as marsh mallow root, nettle, or red clover. Evening primrose oil capsules may improve skin health.

Naturopathy

To flush out the body, drink plenty of water (at least eight glasses a day). The nutrients that particularly benefit the skin are zinc (found in seafood, poultry, and grains), vitamins A and C (in yellow fruits and vegetables and leafy greens), the B vitamins (in lugumes, eggs, and whole grains), and omega 3 fatty acids (in oily fish). Avoid or take in moderation drinks that contain alcohol or caffein. Also, applying to the skin a cloth soaked in milk will help soothe dryness and itchiness. Leave it in place for a few minutes, then rinse.

WARTS

Small, hard growths of flesh, known as warts, are caused by the human papillomavirus. The most common type of wart usually occurs on the hands or the knees. Plantar warts are flat, inward-growing warts that appear on the soles of the feet. Warts also occur on the genitals—if you have genital warts, see a doctor, because they are transmitted sexually and are associated with an increased risk for cervical

WARNING

Precancerous growths may sometimes be mistaken for warts. If you have a growth on the skin that enlarges, darkens, or bleeds, consult your doctor.

VIOLET DECOCTION FOR INFLAMED SKIN

A folk remedy for sore skin is a decoction of violets. The leaves, stems, and flowers have anti-inflammatory properties and may soothe irritation. Add ¼ cup of dried violets to 4 cups of cold water. Cover and heat slowly. Remove the liquid from the heat as soon as it boils. Let it stand for 15 minutes, then strain through cheesecloth.

USING THE DECOCTION
Drink 4 fluid ounces (½ cup) before meals or apply the liquid in a compress to the affected skin twice a day.

cancer. Although warts can sometimes disappear on their own within days, they can also last for months or years. Conventional treatments include applying over-the-counter plasters, lotions, and ointments, burning with chemicals, cauterizing with an electric needle, or freezing with liquid nitrogen. Some people swear by herbal and folk remedies for warts—homeopathy may be helpful, too.

Herbalism

Tea tree, because it has antiviral capabilities, is recommended by some herbalists for treating warts. Apply a little oil or cream to the wart morning and night, but discontinue the applications if they cause irritation. An herbalist may also advocate applying an ointment that contains bloodroot or the juice of fresh celendine leaves. Garlic also has antiviral properties; simply crush a fresh clove and bind it to the wart with gauze, but shield the surrounding skin, because garlic may cause irritation.

Folk remedies

Crush an onion to extract the juice, and apply the onion juice to the wart daily for 20 days, or apply milkweed milk (latex) to the wart daily until it disappears.

Homeopathy

Thuja For warts that are large or cauliflower shaped.
Natrum muriaticum For warts on the palms of the hands, when the palms are hot and sweaty.

BOILS

When a hair follicle becomes infected, the skin may become inflamed and a pus-filled boil may develop. Boils are most common in the armpits and on the groin, thighs, buttocks, and the back of the neck. Recurrent

Slippery elm poultice for boils

Mix 10 ounces of powdered slippery elm with enough boiling water to make a paste. Allow the paste to cool slightly, spread it over the boil, and cover with a piece of gauze. Leave the paste until it is completely cool. Repeat this procedure every day until the boil has discharged.

Ginger and cinnamon tea to improve circulation

Ginger and cinnamon act as circulatory stimulants. Drink ½ cup (4 fluid ounces) of the decoction three times a day. The liquid can also be used as a hand and foot bath; just quadruple the recipe below and add 8 ounces of Epsom salts. You can make a large amount—the mixture will keep for up to five days.

MAKING THE DECOCTION
Add ½ ounce of sliced fresh gingerroot and ½ ounce of cinnamon sticks to 2 cups of water. Bring to a boil, then simmer for 10 to 15 minutes. Strain and store in the refrigerator.

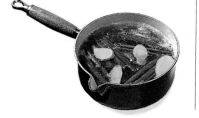

boils may be a sign of weakened resistance to infection due to stress, exhaustion, illness, or an unhealthy diet.

Small boils are usually left to clear up by themselves. If a boil is large and painful, conventional treatment includes oral antibiotics and painkillers and lancing the boil with a needle. Never try to lance or squeeze a boil yourself, since you may spread the infection. In severe cases, a boil may be lanced with a surgical knife, under local anesthetic. It is important that you pay particular care to hygiene when you have a boil—wash your hands before touching food, do not share a towel or washcloth with anyone, and keep the skin around the boil sterile by using an antiseptic soap. Herbalism, hydrotherapy, Chinese herbalism, and naturopathy may prove helpful.

Herbalism

A slippery elm poultice is recommended for drawing out the pus from a boil, and lavender oil or calendula tincture as antiseptics. Other treatments include applying calendula or goldenseal poultices or crushed garlic to the boil. If boils are thought to be caused by lowered immunity, infusions of immune-boosting herbs such as echinacea and garlic are recommended. Echinacea and garlic can also be taken as tablets. Goldenseal may help to promote healing. (Do not take goldenseal if you are pregnant or suffer from hypertension.)

Hydrotherapy

You can help bring a boil to a head by applying alternate hot and cold compresses. Start with a hot compress for three to four minutes and follow with a cold compress for 30 to 60 seconds. Repeat this three to five times. Alternatively, sit in a warm bath that has ½ to 1 pound of Epsom salts added. Do this twice a day until the boil has discharged.

Chinese herbalism

According to doctors of Chinese medicine, boils are caused by Fire Poison in the body. To eliminate this, try cleansing herbs such as Pu Gong Ying (dandelion), Lian Qiao (forsythia fruit), Zhi Hua Di Ding (a type of violet), and Tian Hua Fen (heavenly flower powder mixture).

Naturopathy

If you are prone to boils, a change in your diet may increase your resistance. First, eat lots of green vegetables—they are thought to have cleansing properties. Second, drink

at least eight glasses of water a day (begin the day by drinking a glass of water with the juice of a lemon added). Third, eat lots of zinc-rich foods, such as poultry, fish, liver, and cereals.

COLD SKIN AND CHILBLAINS

When the extremeties are exposed to very cold temperatures, the small blood vessels below the skin constrict; circulation becomes inadequate and the tissue is starved of oxygen. This can result in cold, clammy skin with itchy, purple-red swellings, called chilblains. Children and the elderly are most commonly affected, but the condition can be prevented by keeping feet and hands warm. If chilblains do occur, you can try aromatherapy, herbalism—both Western and Eastern—and hydrotherapy to relieve the discomfort.

Aromatherapy

Massage will increase blood flow to the area of cold skin so that tissues will get enough oxygen. Add three drops of either marjoram or black pepper essential oil to a base massage oil, such as peach kernel, and rub briskly into the skin (do not do this if the skin is broken). To improve circulation, aromatherapists recommend regular body massages and taking baths containing essential oils like rosemary, juniper, or cypress.

Herbalism

Herbalists recommend an infusion or decoction of cayenne, cinnamon, prickly ash, hawthorn, or ginger to improve circulation. External treatments include commercially prepared calendula cream or *Aloe vera* gel applied to skin that is chilled, inflamed, or itchy. Popular folk remedies include rubbing fresh ginger or lemon juice onto the area of cold skin (do not use these remedies if your skin is broken).

Chinese herbalism

Poor circulation and chilled skin are thought to be due to a Blood deficiency; blocked Energy; Cold in the Body; or Yang deficiency (see page 27). Herbs that may be prescribed to nourish the Blood and Energy of the body are Ren Shen (ginseng), Zhi Gan Cao (treated licorice root), Shou Di Huang (treated Chinese foxglove root, also known as pure rehmannia), Huang Qi (astragalus) and Dang Gui (Chinese angelica). To warm the body and move Energy and Blood, Gui Zhi (cinnamon sticks) and Sheng Jiang (fresh gingerroot) may be prescribed.

Alleviating Circulatory Problems with

Aromatherapy Techniques

If you suffer from poor circulation and are prone to cold extremities in the winter months, aromatherapy and massage techniques may help. Stimulating essential oils can warm the skin; massage will encourage blood flow.

Essential oils are aromatic essences distilled or pressed from plant flowers, leaves, bark, berries, and roots. Each oil has its own qualities—some are stimulating and uplifting; others are calming or sedating. The best essential oils for treating circulatory problems are a combination of stimulating oils, like black pepper, and calming oils, such as lavender.

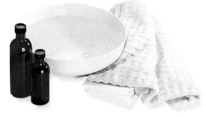

USING ESSENTIAL OILS
Oils can be added to water and applied in a compress, or they can be blended and used for massage.

A FRAGRANT COMPRESS

The feet are particularly affected by circulatory problems, especially among older people whose circulation is more likely to be impaired. Suffering from itchy, red—or even just cold—feet during the winter is extremely common; applying warming essential oils to the feet in the form of a compress can relieve discomfort. Lavender and chamomile oils are soothing and may relieve skin irritation and inflammation; rosemary oil is refreshing and stimulating. Before you apply a compress—or essential oils in any form—make sure that your skin is not broken.

FOOT MASSAGE

Take 3 teaspoons (½ fluid ounce) of a base oil and add three drops of rosemary oil, one drop of black pepper oil, and three drops of lavender oil.

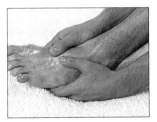 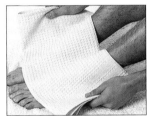

APPLYING THE OILS
Pour the blended oils into your hands and massage your foot using small circular strokes. Then apply brisk rubbing movements to each toe.

WRAPPING THE FEET
When you have completed the massage, wrap your feet in a towel to keep them warm and lie down and relax for 15 minutes.

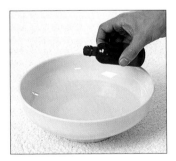 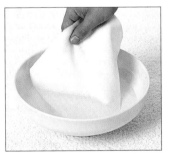

1 *Add 5 to 10 drops of lavender, rosemary, or chamomile oil to one pint of hot water in a bowl. Stir the water until the oil disperses evenly.*

2 *Take a piece of absorbent material and lay it on the surface of the water so that it soaks up the oil.*

3 *Place the compress over the feet and cover with towels. Lie down and relax for 10 to 15 minutes.*

PREVENTING ABSCESSES

According to naturopaths, recurrent abscesses may be from a sluggish digestive system or a compromised immune system. You may need to assess your diet and lifestyle and change both accordingly.

▶ *Reduce the effects of stress in your life—take up meditation or yoga.*

▶ *Increase the amount of liquid you drink (preferably water and herbal teas) to at least eight glasses a day.*

▶ *Avoid refined sugar and flour, alcohol, caffeine, processed foods, fried foods, and dairy products.*

▶ *Eat at least five portions of fresh vegetables and fruits a day.*

GARLIC CURE FOR FUNGAL INFECTIONS Crush 3 cloves of garlic and mix with 3 tablespoons of honey. Apply liberally to the affected area of skin and wrap with gauze.

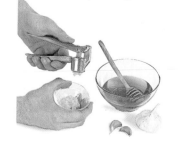

Hydrotherapy

Daily hot and cold showers will help improve circulation. Use hot and cold water alternately for 5 to 15 seconds each and repeat four to six times during each shower. While in the shower, rub your body with a soft brush, always moving toward the heart.

DIAPER RASH

Almost all babies develop diaper rash at some point. The skin, normally covered by the diaper, has pimple-like bumps that may become scaly or crusty. Sometimes the sores ooze and have an unpleasant odor.

Factors that may precipitate the problem include friction, introduction of new foods, skin contact with stale urine, detergent residue in cloth diapers, and chemicals used in some disposable products.

Diaper rash responds very well to natural remedies and good common-sense care. However, a doctor should be consulted if the area becomes red and inflamed, pus-filled sores develop, or if the baby is feverish, listless, or has diarrhea.

The best treatment is to keep the skin dry and exposed to the air as much as possible. To minimize mess, place the baby on a rubber mat covered with a towel. Change the diaper as often as possible and avoid use of plastic pants. After wiping the baby's bottom, you can apply a mild vinegar solution (1 part vinegar to 8 parts water) to neutralize the ammonia that forms in urine. Herbalism may speed healing.

Herbalism

Coat the skin with aloe gel or comfrey ointment. In stubborn cases, applying a poultice of powdered comfrey root might help. Also, using arrowroot powder or cornstarch instead of commercial baby powder is likely to be less irritating to the skin.

COLD SORES

An infection caused by the herpes simplex virus, a cold sore consists of clusters of inflamed blisters around the mouth that burst and crust over. When the virus first strikes it is often accompanied by flulike symptoms and sometimes blisters in the mouth or on the lips. After this initial attack, the virus remains dormant in nerve cells until a specific trigger, such as exposure to sun or cold wind, stress, illness, or poor diet, reactivates it. An outbreak is often preceded by a tingling sensation on the skin.

Cold sores can be prevented or treated using an antiviral drug called acyclovir, either applied to the skin or taken orally. Applying sunblock to your lips before going out in strong sunlight is a good idea. Naturopathy may help to prevent outbreaks.If you do develop a cold sore, try aromatherapy, herbalism, or homeopathy.

Aromatherapy

Aromatherapists recommend tea tree oil for its antiviral properties. Geranium, lemon balm, lavender, bergamot, and eucalyptus essential oils can also help clear up cold sores. Combine 10 drops of any of these oils with $\frac{1}{3}$ fluid ounce (2 teaspoons) of alcohol and apply it to the cold sore whenever you feel the tingling sensation.

Herbalism

Apply a strong tea of lemon balm, myrrh, or goldenseal externally at the first sign of tingling. Ginger juice and fresh garlic may also be effective. To speed healing when the sores break out, mix commercially prepared calendula cream (1 teaspoon) with three drops of tea tree oil (or two drops of lavender oil) and apply to the cold sore. You can also try a tincture or infusion of hyssop. For long-term prevention, take echinacea and garlic to help boost the immune system.

Homeopathy

Natrum muriaticum For cold sores that affect the corners of the mouth and are due to stress or exposure to the sun.
Rhus toxicodendron For cold sores around the mouth.

Naturopathy

Eat plenty of vegetables, fruits, cereal grains, and sesame and pumpkin seeds for general good health. To strengthen the immune system and speed healing, take supplements of vitamin B complex, vitamin C, and vitamin E. Consult a doctor before taking vitamin E supplements if you have heart disease or hypertension.

FUNGAL INFECTIONS

Athlete's foot and ringworm are two of the most common fungal skin infections. Athlete's foot affects the skin between the toes (usually the fourth and fifth toes), which becomes cracked, sore, and itchy. Ringworm can affect the skin anywhere on the body, appearing as red, ring-shaped patches. Sometimes a fungal infection is a secondary problem, as when eczema becomes infected with fungus.

Ringworm and athlete's foot are usually treated with external preparations containing antifungal drugs. For fungal infections of the nails or persistent infections, oral antifungals are used.

Since fungal infections are highly contagious, you should pay careful attention to hygiene. Shower or bathe at least once every day and gently pat your skin dry with a towel. Wear leather shoes and cotton socks. Change your socks frequently.

Herbalism, aromatherapy, and naturopathy may rid the body of fungal infections.

Aromatherapy
Tea tree, lavender, myrrh, patchouli, and geranium essential oils can be used to treat fungal skin infections (avoid myrrh during pregnancy). The oils should be mixed with a base oil (10 drops per tablespoon) and applied to the affected areas.

Herbalism
Herbs such as tea tree, calendula, and thyme are thought to have fungicidal properties. Try mixing two drops of thyme oil with 1 teaspoon of calendula ointment. Or dilute one part of tea tree oil with five parts of calendula oil; apply to the skin.

Naturopathy
Increase your natural immunity to fungal infections by eating plenty of raw vegetables and garlic. The vitamins and minerals that help keep skin healthy are vitamin B complex, vitamin A, vitamin E, and zinc.

ACNE
This is a chronic skin condition characterized by blackheads, whiteheads, pustules, and cysts on the face, neck, and back. Acne involves more than pimples and blackheads, although the same natural therapies can be used to treat both.

The most common cause of acne is inflammation of hair follicles and sebaceous glands due to bacterial infection. Acne may be aggravated by hormonal factors—it is common during adolescence. Some women have premenstrual acne or develop acne in response to taking the contraceptive pill (although others find that the pill brings relief). Occasionally, acne results from an allergy to a chemical, such as a detergent.

Conventional treatments include cleansing the skin thoroughly and applying antiseptics. Antibiotics or other drugs are prescribed for severe cases. Contraceptive pills may be prescribed for some women,

TREATING PROBLEM SKIN
If you have acne, do not squeeze pimples because this will open them to further infection. Wash the skin twice a day with medicated soap. Aromatherapists recommend steaming your face with boiling water to which 2 drops each of lavender, chamomile, and tea tree essential oils have been added.

CABBAGE CURE
Finely chop a cabbage and extract the juice by putting the leaves in a blender or crushing them with a mortar and pestle. Strain and apply the juice to the skin.

and ultraviolet light treatment is occasionally employed. Herbalism and naturopathy may also be useful.

Herbalism
Acne might respond to calendula, which has astringent, anti-inflammatory, and antiseptic properties. Calendula can be applied in two ways: as a lotion made from a tincture or as a face wash made from an infusion mixed with an equal part of witch hazel water or solution. Herbalists prescribe infusions or decoctions of dandelion root and leaf, nettle leaf, and burdock root, which are thought to remove toxins and cleanse the blood. If acne results from a hormonal imbalance, false unicorn root, sage, wild yam, or Chinese angelica may be recommended (avoid sage during pregnancy).

Naturopathy
Cleanse your system by drinking at least eight glasses of water a day and eating five to eight servings of fresh vegetables and fruits. Reduce your intake of dairy products, fried foods, nuts, sugar, bread, red meat, caffeine, and alcohol. Useful dietary supplements are vitamin B complex to decrease sebum (the skin's oily secretion) production, vitamin A to improve overall skin health, vitamin C to fight infection, and vitamin E to prevent scarring. Consult a doctor before taking vitamin E supplements if you have heart disease or hypertension.

URTICARIA
Urticaria, commonly known as hives and also nettle rash, is characterized by itchy wheals (raised pale bumps surrounded by redness) and blisters, usually on the limbs

Traditional cures for urticaria
There are many folk remedies for urticaria (hives), including rubbing slices of onion on the skin, applying cabbage leaf juice as a lotion, or applying the juice of a crushed yellow dock leaf to a nettle sting.

A natural deodorant
Lavender has aromatic properties that can counteract unpleasant body odor. Add 6 drops of lavender essential oil to 2 cups of distilled water. Apply with cotton balls twice a day to the parts of the body that perspire easily.

STORING
LAVENDER WATER
Keep the water in a dark bottle. Light can affect the active ingredients in essential oils.

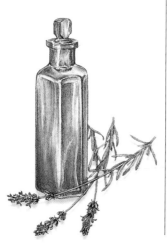

and trunk. It is often a reaction to contact with plants such as stinging nettle, in which case symptoms are usually short-lived. Urticaria can also be caused by an allergy to food, for example, shellfish, strawberries, eggs, or nuts; medications such as aspirin; and food additives like tartrazine (a food colorant). Excessive exposure to heat, cold, or sunlight also may be culprits. Persistent urticaria should be seen by a doctor.

The itching and inflammation of urticaria are usually treated with calamine lotion and antihistamines. In severe cases, a doctor may prescribe a short course of steroids

Herbal medicine and homeopathy can be useful treatments for urticaria. Anti-allergy diets play an important role in the natural treatment of food-related urticaria.

Herbalism
Herbal medicine offers several remedies: calendula cream to soothe the skin, chickweed cream to relieve itching, and chamomile cream or infusion to relieve inflammation. Adding finely ground oatmeal to warm bathwater is therapeutic. You can also try taking evening primrose oil capsules.

Homeopathy
Apis mellifica For urticaria that is accompanied by fever and sweating.
Natrum muriaticum For urticaria that is accompanied by prickly heat.
Urtica urens For red, raised blotches that are better when rubbed and are associated with joint pain.
Dulcamara For a lumpy rash that is made worse by exposure to heat and scratching.
Rhus toxicodendron For a burning, stinging, itchy rash that gets worse in the cold.

Naturopathy
If you suspect that your urticaria is an allergic response to a particular food or food additive, try eliminating it from your diet. It is sometimes necessary to stop eating the problem foods shown on page 66 and then reintroduce them one by one to discover which one causes the reaction.

POISON OAK, IVY, AND SUMAC
Many people react to the oils in these plants by breaking out in an itchy, blistery rash. Prompt action right after exposure may avert or minimize symptoms. As soon as possible, wash all exposed skin with rubbing alcohol or water and laundry or dishwashing liquid. Wearing rubber gloves, remove and launder separately clothing and

shoes that came in contact with the plants. Never burn these plants; their smoke can cause lung inflammation. To ease itching, apply calamine lotion, a paste of baking soda, or cold compresses. A coating of vitamin E oil may reduce inflammation. Herbal remedies can also help.

Herbalism
To minimize rash development, herbalists recommend applying the juice from the leaves or stems of jewelweed (*impatiens capensis*) as soon as possible after exposure. Covering the affected area with gel from an Aloe vera leaf or with crushed plaintain leaves may help ease itching.

EXCESSIVE PERSPIRATION
Heavy perspiration can be a localized problem, involving the palms, the soles of the feet, or the armpits, or it can affect the entire body. If you suffer from whole-body perspiration, consult your doctor to make sure that there is no underlying illness.

Apart from heat and physical activity, causes of excessive perspiration include anxiety, stress, fever, excitement, or menopause.

A doctor treats generalized sweating with drugs that act on the nervous system. Localized sweating may be reduced with an aluminum chloride solution. Acupuncture, herbs, and homeopathy may be helpful.

Acupuncture
Excessive sweating, and menopausal hot flashes in particular, can be treated with acupuncture. Treatment involves toning the kidneys and increasing the body's Energy.

Herbalism
Chlorophyll, which is a substance found in all green plants, is thought to have deodorizing properties. Rubbing fragrant fresh herbs, such as mint, under the arms at least twice every day may help mask perspiration odor.

Homeopathy
Many remedies are intended to reduce sweating, but because sweating has many different causes, it is best to consult a homeopath for diagnosis and treatment.

PSORIASIS

When skin cells reproduce at an abnormally fast rate—up to 10 times as fast as normal in some cases—the result is thickened patches of inflamed skin, often covered with silvery, flaky scales of dead skin. This is psoriasis, and it tends to recur in attacks of varying severity. Psoriasis usually occurs on the knees, elbows, hands, and scalp. Its cause is unknown, although there may be a hereditary factor. Stress, skin damage, illness, or the withdrawal of certain drugs, such as corticosteroids, can trigger an attack.

Ultraviolet light or exposure to moderate sunlight together with ointments helps clear up psoriasis. External antipsoriatic medications include steroids, coal tar creams, and salicylic acid. Drugs to slow down the rate of skin cell division are prescribed.

Chinese herbalism may provide a cure by correcting the bodily imbalances perceived to be the underlying cause of psoriasis. Hydrotherapy may alleviate the condition.

Chinese herbalism

Practitioners of Chinese medicine believe that during an acute attack of psoriasis there is excess Heat in the Blood. They prescribe herbs to cool the blood, such as Tu Fu Ling (greenbrier), Sheng Di Huang (Chinese foxglove, also known as raw rehmannia) and Mu Dan Pi (tree peony root). Since Heat in the Blood over long periods of time can be damaging, Blood herbs such as Dang Gui (Chinese angelica root) and Shou Di Huang (prepared Chinese foxglove root, also known as pure rehmannia) are prescribed. Alternatively, if the Blood has become "stuck" or has stagnated, stimulating herbs such as Chuan Xiong (lovage root) or Tao Ren (peach kernel) are recommended.

Hydrotherapy

Take a dip in the ocean to reduce a severe attack of psoriasis. Alternatively, take a daily bath at home, with water at body temperature and 1 pound of sea salt added. This is relaxing and can help during the acute phases of the disease. Sufferers may find that regular saunas are helpful, or hot compresses applied to the affected areas.

ECZEMA

A common inflammatory skin condition, eczema is characterized by itching, redness, scaling, weeping, blistering, and bleeding. There are various types of eczema: atopic eczema, which occurs in people with an

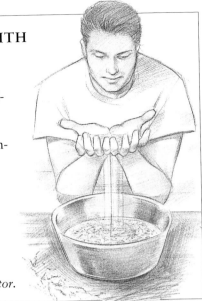

TREATING PSORIASIS WITH CHINESE HERBALISM

In Chinese medicine, the herb Ce Bai Ye (arborvitae) is recommended as a treatment for psoriasis. It comes from an evergreen conifer and is thought to have anti-inflammatory properties. To make a wash, add ½ ounce of Ce Bai Ye to 2 cups of water. Simmer the mixture for 30 minutes.

APPLYING THE SKIN WASH
Bathe the skin in a decoction of Ce Bai Ye in the morning and at night. Store any unused wash in a refrigerator.

inherited tendency to allergies; nummular eczema, which affects any part of the body and resembles ringworm; stasis eczema, affecting people with varicose veins and poor circulation in the legs; and hand eczema, which appears as itchy blisters on the palms of the hands.

Doctors prescribe steroid preparations to reduce inflammation, antihistamines to relieve itching, and antibiotics for infection. Calamine lotion is soothing, and emollient creams reduce dryness.

Western and Chinese herbalism may help eczema. Naturopathy stresses eliminating foods that may cause allergies or sensitivities.

Chinese medicine

Both Chinese herbs and acupuncture are intended to remedy the disharmonies or imbalances associated with eczema (see page 56).

Herbalism

Apply commercially prepared chickweed cream for intense itchiness and calendula cream for dryness. Try adding finely ground oatmeal to your bathwater or use oatmeal soap. Drinking a nettle infusion may cleanse the system.

Naturopathy

Simplify your diet to see if your eczema is diet related. Eat basic foods—brown rice, beans, and vegetables—and then add other foods one by one to see which, if any, aggravates the eczema. Common culprits are dairy products, tomatoes, strawberries, citrus fruits, red meat, shellfish, wheat, spicy food, beer, red wine, processed foods, and refined sugar.

AN OATMEAL BATH
Oatmeal may soothe sore, inflamed, or irritated skin. Put 1 cup of oatmeal in a cheesecloth bag, attach it to your bathtub faucets, and let the warm water run through it. Or you can add 1 or 2 cups of finely ground oatmeal directly to the bathwater.

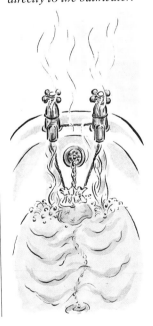

The Chinese Herbalist

Herbal medicine has been practiced in China for thousands of years and is part of an ancient healing system that also includes acupuncture, exercise, massage, and diet. Some skin problems often respond to treatment with Chinese herbs.

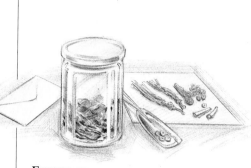

EXOTIC HERBS
Chinese herbal remedies look different from Western ones. Whereas Western herbalists usually recommend plant leaves, flowers, or roots, a Chinese herbal remedy could contain ingredients as diverse as cicada shells or fungus root.

Chinese medicine does more than simply treat a symptom—a traditional Chinese practitioner considers the health of your whole body.

How does Chinese herbal medicine differ from Western medicine?
Rather than looking for a single cause of a disease, a practitioner will search for imbalances or disharmonies, for instance, the flow of vital energy, or *chi*, in the body may be blocked. Herbs are prescribed to correct the balance or re-create harmony.

How do herbalists make assessments?
A practitioner of Chinese medicine establishes the nature of your disharmony through questions and observation. Before recommending a

remedy, he or she builds up a detailed picture of symptoms, medical history, lifestyle, diet, sleep patterns, emotions, and behavior. The practitioner listens to your voice, observes your skin color and texture, looks at the color and coating of your tongue, and takes the pulse at your wrist to establish its rhythm and strength.

What do Chinese practitioners think is the cause of eczema?
An acute attack of eczema, with a red, raised, and angry rash, is usually considered to be due to Damp-Heat (see page 27) in the body. This can result from stress or overindulging in hot, spicy, and greasy foods, processed foods, and dairy products. Other causes include smoking and drinking alcohol and caffeinated beverages.

Eczema that remains after an acute attack subsides may be attributed to Spleen deficiency, which results in excess Damp in the body. This can be caused by fatigue, eating irregularly, or consuming greasy, sweet, or raw foods or dairy products.

The cause of chronic eczema may be diagnosed as one of three main disharmonies or imbalances—Heat in the Blood with Fire in the Heart; Blood deficiency with Wind and Dampness; or Yin deficiency with Dampness. Often people have not just one, but several different dishar-

RECOMMENDING HERBS
A practitioner of Chinese medicine will recommend herbs in their "raw" state for you to boil as a decoction at home.

Origins

The Yellow Emperor's Classic of Internal Medicine is considered to be the most important ancient text on Chinese medicine. Written at least 2,500 years ago, it represents the first attempt to codify this Eastern system of health and healing.

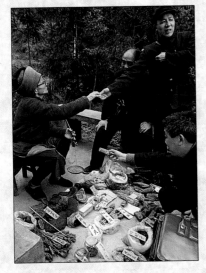

ANCIENT MEDICINES
Many of the herbs prescribed for therapeutic purposes in ancient times are still used in modern China.

monies—an herbalist will provide a remedy suited to the individual.

Which herbs are usually prescribed for eczema?

For Damp-Heat, a common prescription is Long Dan Xie Gan Tang (Chinese gentian root drain the liver decoction). For a Spleen deficiency and excess Damp, herbs such as Fu Ling (a fungal root) or Chen Pi (dried orange peel) may be prescribed. For Heat in the Blood and Fire in the Heart, herbs are given to cool the Blood and expel Heat and Fire. These include Shi Gao (gypsum) and Sheng Di Huang (Chinese foxglove root, also known as raw rehmannia).

If you have Blood deficiency with Wind and Dryness, herbal formulas such as Si Wu Tang or four-substance decoction may be prescribed.

For Yin deficiency and Dampness, an herbalist may recommend yin tonics such as Bei Sha Shen (root of the beech silver top). The herbs shown at right are used to treat eczema.

How are Chinese herbs taken?

A prescription may contain 10 to 15 different herbs. You will be given the dried herbs and asked to boil them at home, since this is the most effective way of taking them. Some are also available as powders, pills, capsules, pastes, ointments, or creams.

Chinese herbal remedies are not necessarily plants. Some contain such minerals as amber or gypsum, or animals like earthworms and seahorses.

Can anyone take Chinese herbs?

Most people can take Chinese herbs. Anyone who is pregnant, elderly, or taking prescribed medicines, should seek conventional medical help first. Chinese herbs have been used for thousands of years and the vast majority are safe, but a few are known to be toxic. Fu Zi (treated aconite root) is banned in the United Kingdom but not in North America, and Ma Huang (ephedra) should be used in relatively small doses; several deaths in the U.S. have been attributed to this herb. Because some herbs may be toxic to the liver, Chinese herbalists may take blood samples to assess any possible danger.

How quickly do the herbs work?

There will probably be an improvement within two to four weeks but you should take the herbs for at least three months to benefit fully.

Can Chinese herbalism be used as a self-help therapy?

Unlike such remedies as essential oils, homeopathic pills, and Western herbs, you cannot buy Chinese herbs over the counter. They are usually available only from practitioners of Chinese medicine, mainly because the diagnostic procedures used are highly specialized and it is thought that each person should have a personalized prescription.

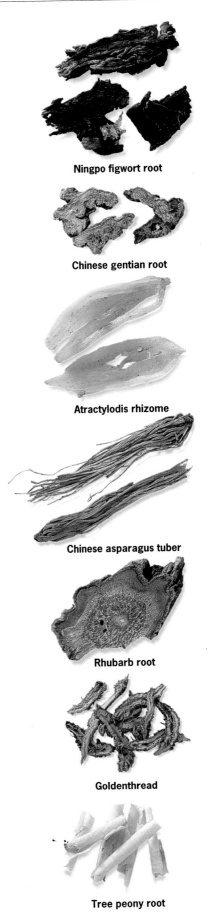

Ningpo figwort root

Chinese gentian root

Atractylodis rhizome

Chinese asparagus tuber

Rhubarb root

Goldenthread

Tree peony root

THE HAIR AND NAILS

Hair and nail conditions can reveal a lot about your general well-being. A lackluster appearance is usually a sign of underlying health problems that may respond to natural remedies.

Some nail problems may be prevented with a healthy diet and by avoiding harsh detergents. Such conditions as head lice may be unavoidable but can be controlled with natural remedies.

DANDRUFF

A common condition in which dead skin is visibly shed from the scalp, dandruff leaves white flakes on the hair and clothes. The usual cause of mild dandruff is a dry scalp. Severe dandruff may be due to seborrheic dermatitis—a scaly, itchy scalp rash.

The usual treatment for dandruff is washing the hair with a dandruff shampoo. If this does not solve the problem, your doctor may prescribe a steroid cream or lotion. If a fungal infection is the underlying cause, the scalp should be treated with an antifungal medication.

Natural therapies for dandruff include aromatherapy to improve blood circulation, herbalism to cleanse the body, and a healthy diet to nourish the scalp.

Aromatherapy

Massaging the scalp with essential oils increases blood circulation and improves the condition of the scalp. For the oils to use and instructions on how to use them, see opposite page.

Herbalism

Dandruff may indicate that the body needs cleansing to improve the skin's health. Cleansing herbs include stinging nettle and red clover leaves taken as a standard infusion. The root of the stinging nettle is another traditional remedy, but rather than taking it internally, it is applied to the scalp as a rinse after shampooing. Some herbalists also advocate applying eucalyptus oil to the scalp. Many herbal rinses for dandruff have been developed over the years. In addition to the ones on the opposite page you might try an infusion of comfrey or add a few drops of the tincture to your shampoo. A few drops of teatree oil added to shampoo may also work. Taking evening primrose oil capsules is recommended for reducing scalp dryness.

Naturopathy

Improve overall health with a diet that includes at least five servings of fresh fruits and vegetables a day. Avoid or cut way down on sugar, white flour, caffeine, and saturated fats from meat and dairy products. You might also try supplements of flaxseed oil—three or four capsules a day.

HEAD LICE

As the name suggests, head lice live on the human scalp where they feed on blood. They leave tiny red, itchy spots that can become inflamed and even infected. The females lay a daily batch of tiny pale eggs, or nits, that are attached to the hairs at the point where they emerge from the scalp. These eggs hatch after seven days. Adult lice can live for several weeks.

Washing your hair with a shampoo that contains lindane or pyrethins is the recommended way to kill head lice and nits rapidly. If you use a shampoo containing lindane, apply it to the scalp and leave it on for 4 minutes; pyrethin shampoos should be left on for 10 minutes. You may need to repeat the treatment after one week. Topical antibiotics are used for scalp infections that arise from excessive scratching.

Aromatherapy and homeopathy are two natural therapies to be used in conjunction with conventional treatment.

Aromatherapy

Bergamot, camphor, eucalyptus, geranium, and lavender essential oils may prevent head lice infestation or eliminate it. Three or four of these oils in combination are recommended by aromatherapists. Mix 5 to 10 drops of each oil with 4 fluid ounces

CLEANSING HERBS FOR DANDRUFF Drinking a standard infusion of red clover and nettle may help clear dandruff by improving overall skin health.

Alleviating Dandruff with

Herbal Remedies

The buildup of dead skin on the scalp may be from infrequent brushing, poor blood circulation in the scalp, overuse of alkaline hair products, or an unhealthy diet. Natural shampoos can help tone the scalp and get rid of dandruff.

There are numerous natural remedies to improve the condition of the hair and the scalp—dandruff in particular may respond to herbal treatments. If you have dandruff, try rinsing the hair with diluted lemon juice (add 2 tablespoons to 2 cups of water). Rinse again with warm water.

Rosemary is an herb that is widely used for toning the scalp—it has astringent properties and it makes the hair shiny. You can use either a standard infusion of rosemary as a hair rinse (follow by rinsing with water), or you can soak 10 ounces of fresh rosemary in 2 cups of ordinary shampoo for two weeks and use the resulting mixture to wash the hair. For an itchy scalp, apply calendula cream. Wash out after 30 minutes.

Soap bark shampoo
Shampoo made from soap bark has cleansing and anti-inflammatory properties. Make a soap bark decoction and mix it with baby shampoo (2 cups to 1 cup).

Essential oils
Rubbing oils into the scalp will improve circulation and give you a healthy scalp. Use vitamin E oil or bay, rosemary, and cedarwood essential oils (five drops each) in jojoba oil (2½ fluid ounces, or ⅓ cup).

Alternatively, try mixing sage oil with olive oil (1 part to 10) and massage into the scalp twice weekly, leaving it on for two hours before rinsing. If you suffer from an itchy scalp, apply cold-pressed linseed oil. Leave it on your scalp overnight and wash out in the morning.

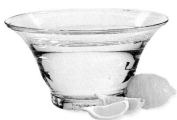

LEMON RINSE
A lemon juice solution is one natural remedy for clearing up dandruff. Follow it with a clear warm water rinse.

DANDRUFF HERBAL SHAMPOO
Blend nettle root, sage, and rosemary for an herbal dandruff treatment.

▶ *Mix ½ ounce nettle root, ½ ounce fresh sage leaves, and 1 ounce fresh rosemary leaves.*
▶ *Add five drops of tea tree oil, 1 ounce baby shampoo, ½ cup methylated alcohol, and 1½ cups water to the herbal mixture. Allow the mixture to infuse for two weeks (shake every day).*
▶ *After two weeks, strain and use as a shampoo two or three times a week.*

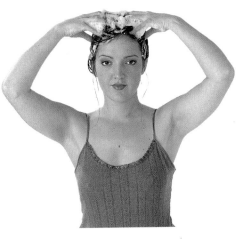

RINSING WITH ROSEMARY
Pour a standard infusion of rosemary over the head to help tone the scalp.

MASSAGING IN ESSENTIAL OILS
Add rosemary, bay, and cedarwood oils to a base oil, apply to the scalp, and leave for 20 minutes before washing out.

SHAMPOOING WITH SOAP BARK
Make a standard decoction of soap bark, mix it with baby shampoo, and use to wash the hair.

59

(½ cup) of a carrier oil, such as almond or hazelnut, then massage into the hair and scalp and leave on for several hours or overnight. Cover your head with a towel or place an old towel on your pillow. As with conventional treatments for head lice, wash out the essential oils using a mild shampoo and then comb the hair using a fine-tooth comb. Repeat this procedure every two days for a week, so that all the lice and nits are eliminated.

Homeopathy

Staphisagria For head lice with a moist discharge on the scalp.

Sulfur For head lice with a dry scalp.

SPLIT AND BROKEN NAILS

The most common causes of weak, split, and broken nails are damage from daily wear and tear, prolonged immersion in water, overuse of polish removers, and a diet that lacks one or more vitamins and minerals. Nail biting also makes them weak and brittle. Occasionally nail problems are a symptom of skin diseases such as psoriasis, fungal infections, and chronic dermatitis. Problems can also occur as a result of heart disease, thyroid disorders, iron-deficiency anemia, malnutrition, or chemotherapy.

If you have split and broken nails, massage moisturizing cream, especially one that contains almond oil, into them regularly, including the cuticles. Always wear rubber gloves when doing household tasks or gardening. Also keep your fingernails relatively short, and when using a nail file or emory board file in one direction only.

Split and broken nails do not require medical attention unless you feel unwell and suspect that they indicate an underlying illness. Hand and finger exercises may help strengthen nails by promoting better circulation, but healthful dietary habits provide the best long-term natural remedy.

Naturopathy

Nails are composed of keratin, the same hard protein that forms the outer layer of skin, hair, and animal hooves. To maintain healthy growth and strength, they need a steady supply of the high-quality protein obtained from meat, fish, chicken, dairy products, and the combining of grains and beans.

If you have thin nails, biotin, a member of the vitamin B complex, may help to improve their thickness. Good sources of biotin are nuts, brewer's yeast, peanut butter, cauliflower, and egg yolks.

Soft, spoon-shaped nails that curve upward are caused by an iron deficiency. Foods rich in iron include red meat, liver, dried beans, whole grains, and green leafy vegetables. To help absorb the iron from plant sources, eat citrus fruits and other foods rich in vitamin C.

HAND EXERCISES TO IMPROVE NAIL HEALTH

The strength of nails depends partly upon the blood supply to the nailbeds. You can improve the blood supply by doing daily hand exercises and massage. Even simple activities such as typing, playing the piano, or drumming your fingers on a tabletop can be extremely effective. Stretching movements are also useful: try grasping the fingers of one hand with the other, or squeeze and push the fingers back over the wrist until you feel a stretching sensation in the palm of your hand and your lower arm.

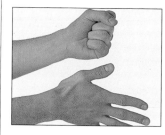

HAND STRETCHES
Open and close your hands quickly—stretching them and then clenching your fist tightly. Do this 10 times every day.

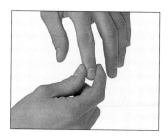

FINGER PULLING
Relax one hand and then wiggle and pull each finger of this hand with the other. Do the same on your other hand.

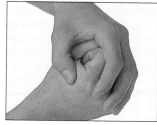

FIST SQUEEZING
Close one hand in the other and squeeze the fingers tightly. Do this five times and then change hands.

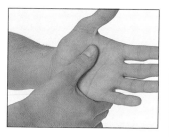

PALM MASSAGE
Massage the palm of one hand with the thumb of the other. Then change hands. Finish by loosely shaking both hands.

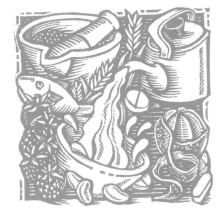

CHAPTER 4

DIGESTIVE PROBLEMS

*Although many people turn to
over-the-counter remedies for indigestion
if they experience discomfort after eating, there
are herbal teas, acupressure points, and relaxation
techniques that can bring relief as well. Also, a
natural therapist may examine diet and eating
habits for an underlying cause of the difficulty.
If the problem is more serious, such as a food
allergy or diverticulitis, a naturopath may
be able to recommend a therapeutic diet.*

APPETITE AND STOMACH PROBLEMS

Everyone suffers from occasional appetite and digestive upsets. Often such problems can be treated successfully by paying close attention to diet and turning to natural remedies for relief.

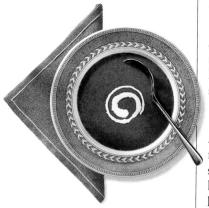

NATURALLY NUTRITIOUS
Soup provides essential fluids and nutrients and will help maintain your health and strength when your appetite is poor.

Poor eating habits—such as gulping down meals or overindulging in food or drink—can cause troublesome symptoms. Careless preparation and poor kitchen hygiene may result in potentially serious food poisoning.

POOR APPETITE

Appetite—the desire to eat—is a sensory response to particular foods. Hunger and satiety, however, are feelings related to the body's need for food, and are regulated by hormones. Together, appetite, hunger, and satiety work to ensure that you get the amount of fuel you need to keep going.

There are many commonplace reasons for poor appetite, such as fatigue, anxiety, or "feeling under the weather." Nasal congestion may affect your appetite by inhibiting your senses of smell and taste and making eating less pleasurable.

Some drugs, such as metronidazole (an antibiotic) and those used in chemotherapy, may reduce appetite, but it should return when the treatment is complete. Poor appetite may occasionally be a symptom of serious illness, such as liver disease or cancer.

See your doctor if your diminished appetite is persistent, has no identifiable cause, or if you have additional symptoms, such as nausea. In the meantime, naturopathy and relaxation may be helpful.

Naturopathy

If you can't eat a "proper" meal, drink nutritious fruit milkshakes or eat vegetable soups to stay healthy.

Research has shown that a deficiency of zinc may reduce appetite, so supplements may be helpful. However, although low doses (12 to 15 milligrams) of zinc are considered to be safe, you should not take zinc supplements without consulting your doctor. Taking too much zinc or taking zinc for long periods may be dangerous.

Relaxation

If anxiety or stress is depressing your appetite, take a lavender essential oil bath, give yourself a foot massage (see page 51), practice deep breathing or yoga, or go for a walk or a swim to relax.

INDIGESTION AND HEARTBURN

Typically, the symptoms of indigestion arise after a heavy meal and include nausea, flatulence, and bloating. Heartburn, the sensation of acidic burning in your stomach or chest, is sometimes brought on by lying down after a large meal.

Eating too much too quickly can cause indigestion or heartburn, and some people find that specific foods consistently upset their stomachs. Coffee, tea, alcohol, and chocolate are common offenders.

Indigestion may be a symptom of a food intolerance or a medical condition such as gastritis (an inflammation of the stomach lining), hiatal hernia (in which part of the stomach protrudes through the diaphragm), or acid reflux (a backwash of stomach acid into the esophagus). Stress, smoking, and certain medications can also cause distress.

Although indigestion may be very uncomfortable, pain should not be a frequent symptom—if you are suffering from stomach pain, weight loss, vomiting, or persistent diarrhea or constipation, see your doctor. Otherwise, herbal remedies and dietary changes may help.

Herbalism

For indigestion or heartburn, drink a standard infusion of either chamomile or fennel, or take slippery elm bark (see page 65).

Naturopathy

Avoid indigestion and heartburn by eating regular meals that are easy to digest, chewing food thoroughly, and taking time between mouthfuls. Reduce your caffeine intake and avoid eating within two hours of going to bed. If you smoke, stop. Adopt simple stress-reduction routines, such as deep breathing, yoga, or tai chi.

STOMACH PAIN

Although it is a symptom of many illnesses, some of the most common causes of stomach pain include ulcer, flu, allergy, gastroenteritis, food poisoning, and gallstones. More often, however, pain is the result of stress, anxiety, or overeating. Occasionally, stomach pain may herald more serious diseases.

Sharp, sudden, severe, or persistent stomach pain should be carefully monitored. If it is accompanied by persistent headache, sweating, pallor, light-headedness, bloody stools, diarrhea, or vomiting, see your doctor.

The treatment of stomach pain depends on its cause, so it is important to obtain a medical diagnosis. Herbalism, acupressure, naturopathy, and relaxation can be used to help alleviate stomach pain.

Herbalism

Chamomile and peppermint teas, or an infusion made from ginger or sage, may help to soothe stomach pains. (Pregnant women should not use sage.) Slippery elm bark mixed with a little water may also be helpful (see page 65).

Acupressure

The points CV 6 and CV 12 may help relieve stomach pain (avoid CV 12 if you have an inflammatory condition of the stomach such as an ulcer). Apply gentle pressure for about two minutes. St 36 (see page 128) may soothe stomachache and indigestion—apply pressure to the point four finger widths below the kneecap, toward the outside of the shinbone.

Naturopathy

Your stomach can stretch to accommodate roughly 6 cups of food or liquid at each meal, but to avoid discomfort you should eat much less than this. If possible, try to eat several small meals throughout the day, rather than one large meal in the evening. If pain results from eating a particular food, eliminate it from your diet and give your digestive system time to recover. Always chew your food thoroughly.

Relaxation

Stress-related stomach pain may respond to moderate exercise such as swimming, walking, or dancing. Meditation, yoga, and tai chi can also help.

NAUSEA

Characterized by the feeling of needing to vomit, nausea is often accompanied by pallor, sweating, dizziness, stomach cramps or pain, or light-headedness. Nausea is frequently associated with indigestion; it can also be a symptom of food poisoning or an infection. Stress, migraine, inner ear disorders, and motion sickness can cause nausea. The first months of pregnancy are notorious for morning sickness, which can occur at any time, not just mornings. Some drugs also induce nausea.

Nausea is usually short-lived and is not a cause for immediate alarm. You should, however, consult a doctor if an attack is persistent—48 hours or more—or if you have persistent diarrhea and vomiting.

Nausea is a symptom rather than an illness, so a doctor will treat the underlying condition. Sometimes, antiemetic drugs may be prescribed. Aromatherapy, herbalism, homeopathy, and acupressure may ease nausea. Some herbs, such as goldenseal and black cohosh, should be avoided during pregnancy; ginger tea and acupressure are the safest remedies for morning sickness.

Aromatherapy

Nausea may be relieved with a drop of undiluted peppermint oil on the tongue. For stress-related nausea or fatigue, a warm bath with four to eight drops of sandalwood or lavender oil added to it may give relief.

Herbalism

Chamomile, peppermint, or ginger tea may calm the stomach. To prevent motion sickness, take one or two ginger capsules 30 minutes before traveling. For stress-induced nausea, drink an infusion of black horehound.

continued on page 66

Acupressure for stomach pain

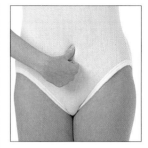

PRESSURE POINT CV 6
This is on the central line of the torso, two finger widths below the navel.

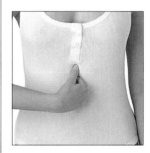

PRESSURE POINT CV 12
This is on the central line of the torso, four finger widths above the navel. Avoid if you have a stomach inflammation, such as an ulcer.

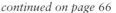

CHAMOMILE INFUSION TO CALM THE STOMACH
Chamomile is one of several herbs that may relieve nausea.

The Herbalist

Herbalists use some of the same diagnostic techniques that conventional doctors do, but they prescribe herbs instead of drugs. Remedies may be in the form of creams, pills, or tinctures; or you may be given dried herbs to infuse at home.

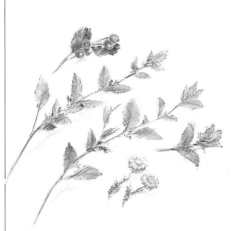

HERBS TO TREAT INDIGESTION
Hawthorn berry, chamomile, lemon balm, and mint have soothing properties that help to relieve indigestion.

Treatment with herbs aims to restore what herbalists describe as the "vital force"—the body's regulating and healing mechanisms. In order to do this, an herbalist will always try to find the source of your illness.

How does herbalism work?

Like conventional drugs, medicinal plants contain pharmacologically active ingredients that affect the body. For example, willow bark contains salicylic acid, the basis for aspirin, whereas foxglove contains digitalis, the basis for the well-known heart drug digoxin.

EXPLORING STOMACH PROBLEMS
After you have described your symptoms, an herbalist will gently palpate the whole of the abdominal area to reveal any areas of tenderness.

One difference between conventional medicines and herbs is that medicine is much more concentrated. Whereas drugs contain one or two active substances, plants may contain a large number, and herbalists claim that these work to greater effect together than they would individually. Thus, the dose of any one substance is relatively low. Herbs are therefore much gentler and generally do not produce the unpleasant side effects that many drugs do. For intance, antibiotics are very efficient at destroying the bacteria that cause infections, but at the same time they destroy the "friendly" bacteria that protect the body from conditions such as thrush.

Plant antibiotics, such as garlic and echinacea, are not as powerful as their synthetic counterparts, but they may help strengthen the body's immune system, increasing resistance to infections in the long term. Herbs tend to encourage the body's own healing systems to work more effectively in addition to acting directly on the disease-causing mechanism.

> **WARNING**
> *Don't exceed the dosage with herbal preparations, and if you suffer side effects, stop treatment. If you have heart disease or hypertension, see your doctor before taking any herbal medicines.*

How does an herbalist make an assessment?

An initial consultation with an herbalist may take up to an hour. The herbalist will ask questions about your diet, lifestyle, and history of illness (and menstrual history for women). If you have a digestive disorder, you will be asked about your eating habits and bowel movements. You may be asked to keep a food diary listing what you eat day by day, along with the symptoms you experience.

Will the herbalist make a physical examination?

Herbalists examine patients using some techniques similar to those of physicians. If you have a digestive problem, palpating the abdominal area will reveal any areas of pain and whether the intestine is too contracted or too relaxed. Blood pressure, pulse, and heart may also be checked.

How do herbalists treat indigestion and heartburn?

An herbalist will propose remedies based on the cause of the indigestion. For a nervous stomach, he may suggest chamomile and lemon balm to help relax and soothe the digestive system. For inflammation and heartburn, an herbalist may recommend marsh mallow and slippery elm to calm the gastrointestinal tract.

If the indigestion or heartburn is due to an irritated stomach lining, licorice may be advised. If the stomach and intestines are overcontracted, then small doses of relaxants like hops or valerian may be useful.

For indigestion accompanied by loose stools, bloating, a weak pulse, and a pale face and tongue, ginger may be advocated. Dandelion root, a mildly bitter remedy, gently improves digestive, liver, and bowel function. For bloating and gas, an herbalist may recommend aromatic herbs—mint, fennel, aniseed, or dill. An herbalist will also give you practical advice about your diet, for instance, drinking less tea and coffee and eating fewer fatty foods.

How quickly should herbal remedies work?

The speed with which herbal remedies take effect depends on the severity of a condition. The longer you have had indigestion, the longer it is likely to be before you are cured. Unlike some drugs, herbs work comparatively slowly, but in doing so, they may provide a more long-term cure. Often, two visits to an herbalist will be enough to treat indigestion.

What training do herbalists have?

In Canada herbalists, also called phytotherapists, are not regulated as practitioners, but some herbal associations do set educational standards. To find a qualified herbalist, contact the Calgary-based Canadian Association of Herbal Practitioners. In the United States there are no training programs or certification procedures for herbalists, but two accredited naturopathic colleges include botanical medicine in their curricula. To find an herbal practitioner or physician who uses herbal remedies, contact: the American Association of Naturopathic Physicians, P.O. Box 20386, Seattle, WA 98102; the American Herbalists Guild, P.O. Box 1683, Soquel, CA 95073; or the American Botanical Council, P.O. Box 201660, Austin, TX 78720.

Origins

Using plants to treat illness is an ancient healing tradition common to all cultures. Knowledge has been passed along for thousands of years from one generation to another. The modern pharmaceutical industry grew out of this herbal tradition, and today some 25 percent of prescription drugs are still derived from plants.

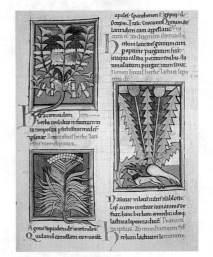

ANCIENT MANUSCRIPTS
Texts dating back to around the 13th century describe the medicinal use of herbs in the West.

WHAT YOU CAN DO AT HOME

To relieve indigestion, make a standard infusion with a combination of chamomile, lemon balm, hawthorn berry, and mint steeped in boiling water for 10 minutes. Drink about one cupful three times a day as needed.

An old folk remedy for heartburn is a mixture of slippery elm bark powder, milk, and water. Slippery elm bark helps soothe the mucous membranes of the stomach and will help alleviate the acidity of heartburn. Combine ½ to 1 tablespoon of the powder with a little water and add 1 cup of milk; take a few teaspoons whenever you are in pain.

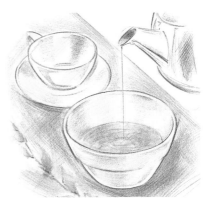

A SOOTHING INFUSION
An infusion of chamomile, lemon balm, hawthorn berry, and mint, will alleviate the discomfort of digestive upset.

Acupressure for vomiting

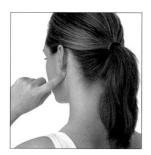

PRESSURE POINT SI 17
This is located in the indentation under your earlobe at the top of your jaw hinge.

FOODS THAT MAY CAUSE PROBLEMS
Among the most common causes of food allergies and intolerances are milk, cheese, eggs, nuts, fish, and shellfish, and gluten grains such as wheat, rye, and oatmeal. Food additives (especially colorants), strawberries, citrus fruits, tomatoes, potatoes, and chocolate also may cause problems.

Homeopathy
Ignatia For motion sickness.
Ipecac For severe, persistent nausea, which is not relieved by vomiting (make sure that you take homeopathic Ipecac—there is an over-the-counter drug available with the same name that induces vomiting).
Nux vomica For nausea that results from overindulgence in food.
Arsenicum album For queasiness accompanied by a burning pain and thirst.

Acupressure
Apply strong pressure to P 6 (see page 133) for one or two minutes. P 6 is on the middle of your forearm, two to three finger widths up from your wrist. Elastic bands that continuously stimulate this point are available.

VOMITING

Vomiting—the violent, involuntary regurgitation of the stomach contents—is commonly due to overeating, too much alcohol, infection, or food poisoning.

Vomiting is usually preceded by persistent nausea and sometimes dizziness, headache, pallor, sweating, or hypersensitivity to smells or flavors. Short-lived episodes of vomiting are rarely serious, but see a doctor if vomiting is persistent; the vomit contains blood; or if vomiting is accompanied by hives or a rash, which may indicate an allergic reaction to a food.

Your doctor may prescribe an antiemetic to stop the vomiting, but natural therapies concentrate on calming the stomach. Since vomiting may cause dehydration, drinking plenty of water after the vomiting has subsided is very important, particularly for children and infants.

Acupressure
Apply firm pressure to P 6 (see page 133) for up to two minutes and breathe deeply. Another useful point is SI 17; apply pressure for two minutes.

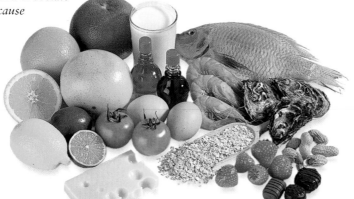

Herbalism
An infusion of ginger helps to soothe stomach upsets. Peppermint tea is also helpful.

Homeopathy
Ipecac For persistent vomiting (take the homeopathic Ipecac, not the identically named over-the-counter drug, which has the opposite effect).
Nux vomica For vomiting due to overindulgence in food or drink.
Arsenicum album For acute vomiting, resulting from eating contaminated food.
Phosphorus For acute vomiting with a craving for cold drinks.

FOOD INTOLERANCES AND ALLERGIES

There are two types of sensitivity to foods: allergies, which are rare and potentially life threatening; and intolerances, which are much more common and less severe. Both food allergies and food intolerances may run in families.

If you are allergic to a food, your immune system reacts as though the food is an invading germ. The symptoms can include rashes, hives, vomiting, and diarrhea. The most serious type of allergic reaction to food is anaphylactic shock, characterized by chest constriction, pulse variations, convulsions, and, finally, collapse.

Food intolerances can cause nasal and sinus congestion, watery eyes, sneezing, wheezing or coughing, headache, and joint or muscle pain. Stomach upsets with bloating, cramping, nausea, heartburn, and flatulence are also common.

If you suspect you have a food allergy or intolerance, you should seek professional medical help. Naturopathy can help prevent recurrences.

Naturopathy
The best approach to food allergies and intolerances is avoidance of the offending food. Record what you eat for a week and monitor how you feel. Your symptoms may be caused by a single item or several in a group—dairy products, for example. If you have symptoms more than twice, regard that food as suspicious. Eliminate it from your diet, then gradually reintroduce it. If you remain symptom-free it is probably not responsible. A naturopath may recommend a true elimination diet in which you reduce your diet to just a few simple foods. This should be done under supervision.

INTESTINAL PROBLEMS

The Western diet tends to be high in refined carbohydrates and low in fiber. This can cause a variety of common problems, such as hemorrhoids, constipation, and diverticular disease, as well as more serious ailments.

Simply increasing the amount of fiber and water in your diet can often prevent intestinal problems in the lower part of the digestive system. Natural therapies such as herbalism and homeopathy may prove helpful in easing discomfort.

FLATULENCE

Excessive gas in the intestines may be accompanied by a distended abdomen, lower abdominal pain, and constipation. The gas is eventually expelled anally.

A high-fiber diet and swallowing too much air while eating are both common causes of flatulence, but it also may result from the food fermenting in the intestines—due to insufficient chewing or constipation. Although uncomfortable and often embarrassing, flatulence is rarely serious. If the problem is persistent or accompanied by pain, however, consult your doctor. The remedies below can be used for quick relief.

Acupressure

Points CV 6 and CV 12 (see page 63) may help relieve gas. CV 6 is located two finger widths below your navel, and CV 12 lies on the central line of the torso four finger widths above the navel. Apply firm, steady pressure to either of these points for two minutes. Avoid CV 12 if you have an inflammatory stomach condition such as an ulcer.

Herbalism

Drinking infusions of ginger, rosemary, or peppermint may relieve gas (avoid rosemary during pregnancy). Alternatively, use these herbs when cooking. Chewing whole cloves or caraway seeds may also help.

Homeopathy

Pulsatilla For gas after eating rich foods, which worsens in the evening and is accompanied by an unpleasant taste in the mouth.

Carbo vegetabilis For a flatulent reaction to fats, meat, or dairy products.

Lycopodium For gas with a craving for sweet things, which worsens in the evening.

Argentum nitricum For flatulence that is worse during menstruation.

COLIC

Characterized by pain that comes in waves, colic is sharp and griping—like a fist being curled and uncurled. The pain of colic is caused by contractions of the affected body part; it is commonly felt as a spasm in the intestine. Causes include stress, food poisoning, infection, kidney stones, gallstones, or other obstructions.

Infantile colic typically affects children two or three months old and tends to occur in the evening. Babies lie with their legs drawn up, cry or scream tirelessly, and resist comforting. They may also have gas. Consult your doctor to exclude other causes of pain or if your baby also has a fever, diarrhea, or constipation.

Babies outgrow colic. For older children or adults, antispasmodic drugs and painkillers may be prescribed. Herbalism, homeopathy, and naturopathy may help but will not have the powerful effect of drugs. If you are in pain, see a physician.

Herbalism

An infusion of fennel, chamomile, or dill seed is recommended to relieve colic. A teaspoonful of the infusion can be given to infants every hour; adults may drink it by the cup.

Homeopathy

Chamomilla For irritable infants, soothed by being carried (ask your homeopath about the correct dosage).

HERBAL INFUSIONS
Give your baby a spoonful of an infusion made with fennel, dill seed, or chamomile to ease the pain of colic.

Acupressure for constipation

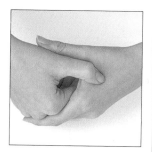

*PRESSURE POINT LI 4
This is located in the
center of the webbing
between the thumb and
the index finger. Avoid
during pregnancy.*

*SALMONELLA
These bacteria, com-
monly found in poultry
and eggs, can cause acute
diarrhea if food is not
handled properly.*

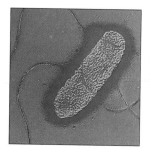

Pulsatilla For babies who are generally
good-natured, who respond well to fresh air,
and who are calmed by gentle rocking (seek
advice from a homeopath about dosage).

Naturopathy
Kidney stones or gallstones can cause colic.
To help prevent these conditions, increase
the amount of fiber in your diet and reduce
your intake of saturated fat (this is found in
foods such as cheese, cream, whole milk,
and meat) and drink at least eight glasses of
water every day.

CONSTIPATION
The normal frequency of bowel movements
varies from person to person—constipation
is characterized by movements that are
uncomfortable or irregular, or by stools that
are unusually hard. Although stress, inactivity, and illness are causes of constipation,
the usual cause is insufficient fiber and
water in the diet.

Consult a physician if you suddenly suffer
from constipation for no discernible reason
and your normal pattern of bowel movements does not return within one week.
Although rare, persistent constipation can
be an early warning sign of disease such as
colorectal cancer.

Many people turn to laxatives to relieve
constipation—ask your pharmacist for
advice. Avoid taking laxatives for long
periods, because you may become dependent on them for regular bowel movements.
The following therapies can help by encouraging the intestines to work more efficiently
or by acting as natural laxatives.

Massage
Although not a cure for constipation, massage may help the intestines contract more
efficiently. Place your fingers on your lower
left abdomen and make small circles using
gentle pressure. Move your fingers one to
two inches up toward your ribs, and massage again. Repeat until you reach your ribs,
then massage across the top of your
abdomen from left to right. Continue massaging inch by inch straight down to your
right hip. Finish by making sweeping clockwise circles over the whole abdominal area.

Naturopathy
To improve bowel function, gradually add
whole grains and more raw or cooked fruits
and vegetables to your meals. Drink eight
glasses of water a day and exercise regularly
for overall muscle tone.

Acupressure
Apply pressure to CV 6, LI 11, Liv 3, or
LI 4. Point CV 6 is two finger widths below
your navel (see page 63). Point LI 11 is at
the outside edge of the elbow crease (see
page 37). Liv 3 is two finger widths up from
the juncture between the big toe and the second toe (see page 131). Do not use Liv 3 or
LI 4 during pregnancy; LI 4 may stimulate
premature contractions.

Herbalism
Some herbs have laxative properties, and,
like conventional drugs, should be used only
for short-term relief. You can try a standard
infusion or decoction of either buckthorn
bark or psyllium.

DIARRHEA
The frequent passing of unformed, watery
stools is known as diarrhea. Common
causes include bacterial, viral, or parasitic
infections; food allergies; a change in food
or water; certain drugs or medical treatments; and stress.

Diarrhea is usually an attempt by the body
to rid itself of harmful toxins, and it will
often clear up on its own. You should, however, consult a doctor if diarrhea continues
for two days or more, or is recurrent; the
stools contain blood; or the sufferer is an
infant or child. You may be prescribed
antidiarrheal drugs and rehydration salts to
replace lost minerals, or antibiotics for a
severe bacterial infection. Natural remedies
are most appropriate for mild diarrhea and
stress-related diarrhea in particular. Try aromatherapy, herbalism, and relaxation, and
drink plenty of water to rehydrate yourself.

Aromatherapy
Use lavender, sandalwood, chamomile, and
juniper essential oils for stress-related diarrhea. You can add 6 to 8 drops of the oils
to your bathwater or inhale the vapors from
a bowl of hot water.

For diarrhea that accompanies a bacterial
or viral infection, take 1 drop each of peppermint and cypress oils on a sugar cube
every two hours, or as required.

Herbalism
Infusions of goldenseal or dill, or a decoction of fenugreek, may be helpful. Do not
use goldenseal if you are pregnant or suffer
from high blood pressure.

Infectious diarrhea in children can be
treated with dill water, made with two
tablespoons of crushed seeds steeped in a

Naturopathy

Naturopaths recommend several steps to improve bowel function: eat plenty of fiber-rich foods, increase the amount of water you drink, follow a cleansing diet, and get the correct exercise.

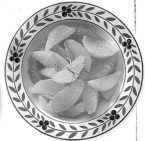

Find out how efficient your digestive system is and whether you need to include more fiber in your diet with a "transit test." This determines how long food takes to pass through your digestive system. At nine o'clock one evening take three charcoal tablets (available from health food stores), or eat strongly colored foods, such as spinach or beets, as "markers." Monitor your stools and note the time when the first significantly darkened stool appears. This should happen within 12 hours of taking the charcoal tablets. Stools should no longer be discolored 24 hours after taking the

charcoal. Any longer would suggest that your bowels are sluggish.

Naturopaths recommend a short cleansing diet to treat constipation. This gives your digestive system a rest and your bowels a chance to empty—avoid this diet if you suffer from diabetes. Alternatively, increasing the amount of fiber in your diet (do this anyway after you have completed the cleansing diet) may be helpful. Dietary changes should be accompanied by moderate exercise—increasing your level of activity and performing specific abdominal exercises can make the intestines more efficient.

ABDOMINAL TONING
Lie on your back and bend your knees with your feet flat on the ground. Lift your hips off the floor and hold for 10 seconds. Repeat five times, twice daily.

THE FOUR-DAY CLEANSING PROGRAM

Simplifying the diet to a few basic foods gives your gut a chance to recover from constipation.
Day 1 Fruit, fruit juices, or mineral water only.
Day 2 Fruit and mixed salads for each meal. Drink mineral water, pure fruit juices, or herbal teas.
Day 3 Fruit and yogurt for breakfast, mixed salad for lunch, and steamed vegetables with cheese for dinner.
Day 4 Fruit or granola with yogurt for breakfast. Salad for lunch and brown rice and vegetables for dinner. Return to normal diet on the fifth day.

ADDING FIBER TO YOUR DIET

The best way to treat constipation is to eat at least two fiber-rich meals and drink eight glasses of water a day. Because fiber cannot be digested by enzymes in the stomach and intestines, it adds bulk and helps waste matter pass through the gut. This relieves constipation.

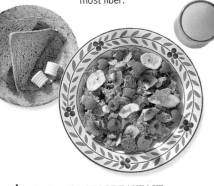

Stone-ground bread contains the most fiber.

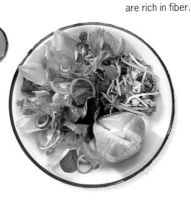

Potato skins are rich in fiber.

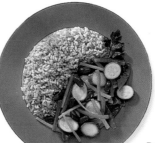

Brown rice contains more fiber than white rice.

A WHOLE-GRAIN BREAKFAST
Eat one slice of whole-wheat bread with a little butter. Follow with a bran cereal with fresh or dried fruit added.

A SALAD AND POTATO LUNCH
Prepare a selection of raw vegetables, flavored with garlic and lemon juice. Eat with a plain baked potato.

A RICE AND VEGETABLE DINNER
Eat brown rice with steamed vegetables and beans or lentils. Have fresh or dried fruit for dessert.

DIARRHEA AND FOREIGN TRAVEL

Diarrhea is very common when visiting foreign countries, especially those with hot climates or poor sanitation. If you become ill, sip bottled water constantly throughout an attack to prevent dehydration. Don't stop eating. This will aggravate dehydration and deprive your body of the nutrients that are necessary for recovery. Although most attacks of diarrhea are short-lived and don't require treatment, you should seek medical help if your stools contain blood or mucus or if the diarrhea is accompanied by fever.

THE DO'S AND DON'TS OF FOREIGN TRAVEL
By following certain rules when traveling in very hot or under-developed countries, you should be able to avoid attacks of diarrhea.

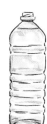

Do drink bottled water and make sure the seal is intact when you buy it.

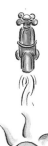

Don't drink local tap water or have ice in drinks.

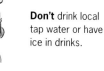

Don't increase your dehydration if you have diarrhea by going out in the sun or overexerting yourself.

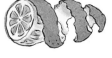

Do eat fruit that you can peel.

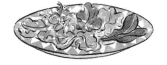

Don't eat salads because the leaves may have been washed in tap water.

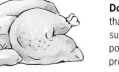

Don't eat foods that spoil quickly, such as meat, poultry, and dairy products.

---

cup of boiling water for 10 minutes and then strained. You should not give your child more than three cups a day.

Relaxation
If diarrhea is due to nervousness or tension, relaxing therapies like yoga may be helpful. For diarrhea that is precipitated by an event such as exams or an interview, practice slow, deep breathing exercises (see page 114) immediately beforehand.

HEMORRHOIDS

Swollen and distended veins in the anal area are known as hemorrhoids or piles; they usually arise from pressure on the lining of the anus. Although there are various causes of hemorrhoids, including pregnancy, they are most often due to constipation. When you strain to pass a stool, the raised abdominal pressure causes the veins of the anus wall to enlarge. Blood pools in these veins and they become abnormally swollen. Hemorrhoids can also be hereditary.

Usually hemorrhoids will appear as brown swellings around the anus, or they can occur inside the rectum. The characteristic symptoms are itchiness, pain when you pass a stool, and bleeding from the anus. The treat-

ment for hemorrhoids depends on the severity of your discomfort. Simply increasing the amount of fiber and water in your diet and trying to keep your bowel movements regular should help prevent hemorrhoids and alleviate symptoms. You can improve your anal hygiene and minimize discomfort by using moistened, unscented, undyed toilet paper to clean the anus after a bowel movement. Over-the-counter creams and suppositories that contain steroids often help relieve the pain and inflammation of hemorrhoids. In severe cases that don't respond to normal treatment your doctor may recommend surgery.

Hydrotherapy can sometimes reduce the uncomfortable swelling and itching of hemorrhoids; herbalism and homeopathy can ease the pain; abdominal massage can help prevent hemorrhoids from occurring in the first place.

HERBAL REMEDIES FOR HEMORRHOIDS
Witch hazel preparations, comfrey ointments, and horse chestnut salves and ointments can be applied to soothe hemorrhoids.

WARNING
Consult a physician if you notice blood in your stools, especially if you have no other symptoms of hemorrhoids. Your physician will be able to rule out the possibility of more serious diseases.

Hydrotherapy
Soaking is recommended to reduce anal swelling. Fill the bath tub with enough warm water to cover your hips, and soak for 20 minutes. You can add 5 to 10 drops of any of the following essential oils: cypress, chamomile, juniper, frankincense, or myrrh (avoid myrrh during pregnancy). Or dissolve a couple of handfuls of Epsom salts in the water; they will constrict the hemorrhoids. Follow your bath with a briefer soak in cool water. Finally, apply witch hazel water or solution to the anal area with a cotton ball.

Herbalism
Astringent herbs, such as pilewort, collinsonia, or witch hazel may relieve pain. These herbs are available as ointments and can be applied to the anal area.

Homeopathy
Berberis vulgaris For tearing, radiating pain, or pain that becomes worse on standing or moving.
Thuja For a stitching pain that is worse when sitting.
Nux vomica For itchiness, pain, and straining to pass a stool.
Sepia For a sensation of having a ball in the rectum and pain that shoots upward.
Sulfur For hemorrhoids accompanied by redness, burning, itching, and oozing.

Massage
If hemorrhoids are brought on by constipation, abdominal massage (see page 68) may help to ease discomfort.

DIVERTICULAR DISEASE
Normally, the lining of the intestines forms a smooth surface along which waste products are carried. Often, pockets called diverticula develop in the intestinal walls. This condition, called diverticulosis, affects more than half of the population of Western countries by the age of 80, but is usually benign and symptom-free. When symptoms are present (in roughly 20 percent of cases) they are similar to those of irritable bowel syndrome (see description, right). They include muscle spasms or cramps in the lower abdomen, mucus in the stools, and diarrhea, constipation, or attacks of both.

Diverticulitis occurs when the diverticula become infected or inflamed. The usual symptoms are fever, intense pain—similar to that of appendicitis—and a rigid, tender abdomen. In a few cases, there may be strictures or abscesses that narrow the intestine's diameter. Consult your doctor if you have any of these symptoms.

Diverticulosis usually responds well to a high-fiber diet, but your doctor may also prescribe a course of antispasmodic drugs. Diverticulitis, on the other hand, should be treated with antibiotics and bed rest. In the small percentage of cases in which abscesses and the risk of gangrene or peritonitis exist, surgery is recommended. Natural remedies for diverticulosis focus mainly on making changes to the diet, but herbs may help relieve discomfort.

Naturopathy
Gradually introduce more fiber-rich foods —beans, fresh fruits, vegetables, and whole grains—into your diet. For the fiber to be effective, you must drink a minimum of eight glasses of water a day. Avoid caffeinated drinks, like coffee, cola, and tea, because caffeine has a diuretic effect and will deplete water in the body. Garlic has antibacterial properties that may help prevent infection. It can be eaten raw, used in cooking, or taken in tablet form.

Herbalism
Powdered slippery elm bark can calm the mucous membranes of the intestines. Mix 1 to 2 teaspoons of the powdered herb with a little water and take a spoonful as needed. Infusions of peppermint or chamomile may also soothe the digestive tract.

IRRITABLE BOWEL SYNDROME
Also known as spastic colon or mucous colitis, irritable bowel syndrome (IBS) is characterized by bloating, flatulence, abdominal pain or cramping, fatigue, and alternating bouts of constipation and diarrhea. Women are more commonly affected than men, and their symptoms may worsen before or during menstruation.

Some natural practitioners think that IBS may be caused by a food allergy, intolerance to dairy products, a yeast infection, excessive alcohol or caffeine intake, or a previous

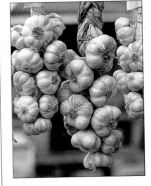

A NATURAL ANTIBIOTIC
Garlic has antibiotic properties that make it useful in preventing some intestinal infections, such as diverticulitis or inflammatory bowel disease. If you are prone to these conditions, try to include plenty of garlic in your diet.

AROMATHERAPY RELIEF
Several essential oils, such as lavender or clary sage, may help to relieve abdominal discomfort. Use the oils in a massage or a compress.

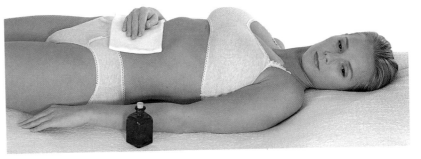

viral, bacterial, or parasitic infection. Anxiety and stress appear often to be contributory factors; however, no definite cause has been established.

For many people, eating more frequent, smaller meals helps alleviate symptoms, as does following a low-fat diet, high in complex carbohydrates and protein.

Aromatherapy, herbalism, homeopathy, Chinese herbalism, and relaxation can ease the discomfort of IBS.

Aromatherapy
For abdominal pain, use essential oils such as black pepper, ginger, lavender, peppermint, orange blossom, and clary sage for relief. Apply them as a massage oil or in a compress on the lower abdomen.

Herbalism
Flatulence, spasms, and cramps can be eased by marjoram, cumin, fennel, cinnamon, peppermint, and thyme (avoid thyme during pregnancy). Enteric-coated peppermint oil capsules, specially prepared to dissolve in the intestines instead of in the stomach, are available at health food stores.

Homeopathy
Aloe For irritable bowel syndrome with mucus in the stools and burning pains.
Argentum nitricum For flatulence, colicky pain, stools containing mucus, and constipation alternating with diarrhea.
Arsenicum album For burning, profuse diarrhea with restlessness, and colic.
Colocynthis For pains that are relieved by warmth, pressure, or doubling over.
Nux vomica For pain relieved by frequent small bowel movements.

Chinese herbalism
The common causes of IBS are thought to be stagnant Liver Energy or a deficiency of Spleen or Stomach Energy. If the main symptoms are abdominal pain and bloating, a practitioner of Chinese medicine may recommend Huo Po (magnolia bark). For constipation, you may be advised to take Dang Gui (Chinese angelica). Fu Ling (poria) may be recommended for diarrhea.

RELAXATION FOR IRRITABLE BOWEL SYNDROME
Yoga offers many relaxing poses that can help ease symptoms of IBS.

Relaxation
If irritable bowel syndrome is caused by stress, any sort of relaxation technique will help. Mild exercise, such as short walks, stretching, tai chi, or yoga, are thought to be particularly effective.

INFLAMMATORY BOWEL DISEASE
Ulcerative colitis and Crohn's disease are similar illnesses that affect the bowel. Symptoms include abdominal pain, nausea, fever, and diarrhea. In ulcerative colitis, stools may contain blood, mucus, or pus; this symptom sometimes occurs in Crohn's disease. The cause of inflammatory bowel disease is unknown, but ulcerative colitis can be associated with stress.

Arthritis is a complication of inflammatory bowel disease. See a doctor if you have pain in your lower back, buttocks, and thighs, aching joints and muscles, unexplained fever, or swollen red patches on your legs.

Orthodox treatment includes anti-inflammatory drugs and steroids for both diseases, but when the condition is severe and does not respond to conventional remedies, surgery may be the only solution. Naturopathy, homeopathy, and herbalism may offer some degree of symptom relief.

Naturopathy
Although the importance of diet in Crohn's disease and ulcerative colitis is disputed by some conventional doctors, naturopaths may suggest that you avoid dairy products and adopt a liquid diet for acute symptoms. When your condition returns to normal, gradually introduce solid food to your diet. This diet, however, should only be followed under medical supervision.

Homeopathy
Mercurius corrosivus For cutting pain, blood or mucus in the stools, and symptoms that worsen in the evening.
Arsenicum album For burning, colic, restlessness, exhaustion, and anxiety that are worse after midnight.
Colocynthis For symptoms that are relieved by hard pressure on the abdomen or by bending over.

Herbalism
To ease inflammation, try taking slippery elm bark. It has mucilaginous qualities and coats the whole intestine. Mix 2 to 3 teaspoons of the powdered herb with water, until you have a mixture that you find palatable. Take between meals.

CHAPTER 5

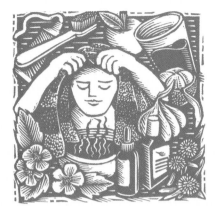

MOUTH, NOSE, AND THROAT COMPLAINTS

*Many common problems that affect the mouth,
nose, and throat are symptoms rather than illnesses.
For instance, a cough may be a symptom of bronchitis,
and nasal congestion may be a sign of influenza or
allergic rhinitis. There are natural remedies to ease
the immediate discomfort of symptoms and
to treat the underlying illness.*

THE MOUTH

The health of tissues in the mouth can be undermined if you eat a lot of sugar, damage them with abrasive substances, or have an illness that has weakened your immune system.

Three helpful natural therapies for treating mouth problems are naturopathy, herbalism, and homeopathy. A naturopath would recommend replacing sugar in the diet with healthy foods, an herbalist would suggest herbs to soothe the mouth or mask bad breath, and a homeopath would prescribe remedies to solve any underlying oral health problem.

HALITOSIS

Bad breath, or halitosis, may stem from certain medications, infections, gum disease, or a stomach disorder, but is most often caused by bacteria in the mouth, smoking, or eating certain foods. You may not notice your bad breath since your sense of smell accommodates itself to persistent aromas and eventually stops perceiving them.

Halitosis is usually worse in the morning. You produce less saliva while you sleep and the resulting dryness produces the odor, which may be increased if you snore or sleep with your mouth open. Brushing your teeth and flossing twice a day is usually sufficient to prevent normal mouth odor, but even good hygiene will not help if bad breath is due to eating pungent foods, such as onions or garlic, drinking strong-smelling beverages like whiskey, or smoking. This is because the odor-causing chemicals in foods, beverages, or tobacco are picked up by the blood and excreted by the lungs when you exhale. Although odors can be masked with mints or cloves, you won't be rid of them until the offending substance leaves your system.

Bad breath that persists despite conscientious brushing and flossing may mean that you have an underlying dental or medical condition. Check with your dentist before seeing your doctor. Herbalism, naturopathy, and homeopathy can mask or help prevent halitosis.

PREVENTING MOUTH AND GUM PROBLEMS

The best way to avoid mouth and gum problems is to brush and floss your teeth twice daily. This will prevent the buildup of plaque— a sticky film of bacteria on the teeth. Plaque contains naturally occurring bacteria (it will form even in the absence of food), and unless it is removed regularly it will cause tooth decay by turning sugar to acid, which then attacks tooth enamel. Accumulated plaque will also weaken gum tissue, which then bleeds easily and can lead to serious gum disease. If you already have gum problems, an infusion of sage can be soothing.

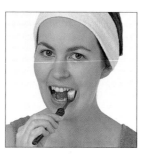

BRUSHING THE TEETH
Holding your toothbrush against your teeth at a 45-degree angle, brush away from the gum edges. Make sure you brush all surfaces of the teeth; this should take at least three minutes.

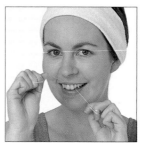

FLOSSING
Press a length of dental floss between the teeth. Gently work the floss down to your gum and then scrape up and down along the side of each tooth. Use a new section of floss each time.

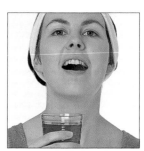

GARGLING
A sage infusion with a pinch of salt makes an excellent gargle; it has antiseptic properties, which makes it good for gum disease, canker sores, and sore throats. Avoid sage in pregnancy.

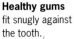

Healthy gums fit snugly against the tooth.

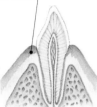

Inflamed gums may cause the gum to retract from the tooth.

THE ORIGIN OF GUM DISEASE
A buildup of hardened plaque, called calculus, traps more plaque, causing gum inflammation and, eventually, loose teeth.

Herbalism

To mask bad breath, chew parsley, a whole clove, or cardamom seeds, or drink an infusion of peppermint or fenugreek seeds (avoid excessive use of parsley during pregnancy). If bad breath is due to a cavity, cloves, which have analgesic properties, may also alleviate pain until you see a dentist.

Naturopathy

Avoid strongly aromatic foods and cut down on refined sugar, which exacerbates tooth decay. If you have a sweet tooth, eat fresh fruits, which contain natural sugar.

Homeopathy

Nux vomica For sour-smelling breath in the morning, or after meals or alcohol.

IRRITATED GUMS

Swollen, tender, inflamed gums—a condition known as gingivitis—are triggered by accumulated plaque between and at the base of the teeth.

Other causes of gingivitis are poor nutrition, especially low levels of folic acid and the B vitamins, ill-fitting dentures, the presence of a local or systemic infection, and cigarette smoking. Specific conditions that create a greater demand for nutrients (particularly folic acid and B vitamins), such as pregnancy or taking the contraceptive pill, may increase the likelihood of gingivitis. Gingivitis is usually painless, but if it is left unchecked, it may lead to a more serious condition called periodontitis, which destroys the bone and tissues that support the teeth. The buildup of plaque can be reduced by proper oral hygiene.

Herbal mouthwashes, homeopathic remedies, and eliminating sugar from the diet may all be effective in promoting healthy gums and alleviating discomfort.

Herbalism

Rinse your mouth several times a day with a standard infusion of sage. You can add five drops of echinacea, myrrh, or rosemary tincture to the infusion, or use the tinctures on their own to make mouthwashes. Avoid sage, myrrh, and rosemary if you are pregnant.

Homeopathy

Mercurius solubilis For inflamed gums, a metallic taste, and profuse salivation.
Phosphorus For gums that bleed easily.
Hepar sulphuris For gums that are painful to touch and that bleed easily, or for abscesses that erupt at the gum line.

Naturopathy

Replace highly refined foods such as cakes, cookies, and doughnuts with whole grains, fresh fruits, and vegetables. Instead of candy and soft drinks, snack on nuts and drink freshly squeezed fruit and vegetable juices. Consult a naturopath to establish whether you would benefit from folic acid, B vitamins, or calcium supplements.

CANKER SORES

Ulcers inside the mouth or on the gums result from viral infections or from injuries, such as an abrasion from a fork or dental brace. They can also be due to a stomach disorder, poor diet, or stress, or they may run in the family.

Canker sores usually clear up relatively quickly. If they persist beyond two or three weeks or if they are accompanied by fever or other symptoms of illness, consult your doctor. The conventional treatment to relieve pain is an analgesic mouth gel applied directly to the ulcer. Herbs and essential oils can be used in mouthwashes to ease discomfort; homeopathic remedies may also bring pain relief.

Herbalism

Add one drop each of geranium oil and lavender oil or a tincture of myrrh to half a cup of water to make a soothing mouthwash (myrrh should be avoided during pregnancy because it's a uterine stimulant).

Aromatherapy

Dilute geranium oil or eucalyptus oil with a base oil and apply as required.

Homeopathy

Arsenicum album For ulcers on the side of the tongue or ulcers that produce a sensation of burning.
Mercurius solubilis For spongy ulcers on the palate or tongue.

AROMATHERAPY FOR CANKER SORES
Add 3 drops eucalyptus essential oil to ½ fluid ounce (1 tablespoon) of a base oil such as sweet almond oil; apply the mixture to the sore.

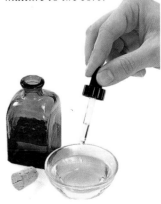

THE NOSE

A nose congested with mucus or blood is uncomfortable and inhibits breathing. Natural therapies can clear the air passages, stop bleeding, or discourage mucus production.

Acupressure for nosebleeds

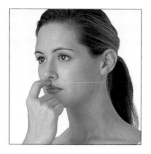

PRESSURE POINT GV 26
This is two-thirds of the way up between your nose and upper lip.

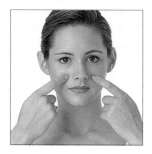

PRESSURE POINT ST 3
This is at the base of your cheekbones above the corners of your mouth.

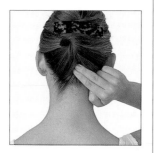

PRESSURE POINT GV 16
This is at the top of your spine in the hollow at the base of your skull.

Nasal problems may take the form of stuffiness and congestion; pain and bleeding from an injury, such as a blow to the nose; an allergic reaction to food, pollen, or pets; or pain and discomfort from inflamed sinuses.

NASAL CONGESTION
The most common causes of nasal congestion are allergic rhinitis, colds (see page 84), and influenza (see page 85). Often, nasal congestion persists even after other symptoms of a cold or flu have gone. A stuffy or runny nose may also be caused by chronic sinusitis (see page 88). Some people experience nasal congestion from tobacco smoke, cold temperatures, or certain foods. This condition, which is called vasomotor rhinitis, is common during pregnancy and when taking oral contraceptives.

Nasal congestion may be characterized by thick, yellow mucus, the constant urge to blow the nose, and breathlessness, or there may be watery secretions. Aromatherapy and homeopathy may help.

Aromatherapy
Inhaling steam from a shower or bowl of very hot water can alleviate congestion. You will get even better results if you add a few drops of an essential oil such as cinnamon, eucalyptus, or peppermint; cover your head with a towel as you inhale. Alternatively, put the oils on a handkerchief and inhale often.

Homeopathy
Kali bichromicum For thick, stringy greenish or yellowish nasal discharge that is difficult to expel.
Natrum muriaticum For copious clear or whitish nasal discharge and a nasal drip.
Nux vomica For nasal congestion at night or outdoors, and a runny nose during the day or when you are indoors.
Arsenicum album For a runny nose that feels congested.

NOSEBLEEDS
The most common causes of nosebleeds are sudden impact, inserting foreign objects into the nose, and blowing too forcefully. The dry air in centrally heated or air-conditioned buildings can increase the risk for nosebleeds. See a doctor if a nosebleed is accompanied by dizziness, drowsiness, nausea, or vomiting; if it lasts for more than 20 minutes; or if nosebleeds recur frequently.

First aid for nosebleeds involves pinching the nose just below the bridge for 10 minutes. Try not to speak, sniff, or spit during a nosebleed, and be sure to rest afterward. Acupressure and homeopathy may help stop the bleeding.

Acupressure
The first-aid point for nosebleeds is GV 26. You can also apply pressure to points St 3, GV 16, and LI 4 (see page 68), which is on the webbing between the thumb and the forefinger (avoid LI 4 during pregnancy).

Homeopathy
Arnica For bleeding resulting from a blow.
Phosphorus For blood that is bright red and slow to clot.
Belladonna For bloody mucus or a nosebleed that is accompanied by a flushed or reddened face.

STOPPING A NOSEBLEED
Tilt your head forward and pinch the fleshy part of the nose just below the bridge.

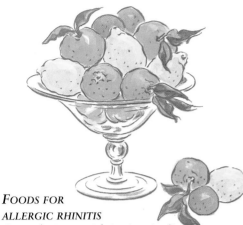

*FOODS FOR
ALLERGIC RHINITIS
Citrus fruits are rich in vitamin C
and bioflavonoids and are particularly
recommended to alleviate allergy symptoms.*

ALLERGIC RHINITIS

Commonly called hay fever, allergic rhinitis is triggered by a sensitivity to seasonal irritants, such as pollen and mold spores, or to omnipresent ones, such as household dust or pets. Hay fever symptoms are like those of a head cold: a stuffed or runny nose, watery eyes, sneezing, wheezing, and fatigue.

Over-the-counter antihistamines can relieve symptoms, but see a doctor if your symptoms are persistent or debilitating. Prescription-strength antihistamines, desensitizing injections, or, in severe cases, cortisone may be recommended. Using air conditioners or air filters in the home may be helpful. Regular vacuuming, damp mopping, and dusting can remove much of the allergen, but dust and pollen will stick to your hair and clothes. Acupressure, aromatherapy, homeopathy, and naturopathy may help relieve symptoms.

Acupressure

Try applying pressure to point Bl 2 (see page 46), found on either side of your nose at the edge of each eyebrow; point CV 6 (see page 63) on your midline two finger widths below your navel; and LI 4 (see page 68) on the webbing between your thumb and forefinger (avoid if you are pregnant). Bl 10 and Kid 27 may also be useful.

Aromatherapy

A few drops of essential oil of lavender combined with 1 tablespooon of a carrier oil may help soothe the nasal symptoms of hay fever. Use it to massage the sinus area.

Homeopathy

Arsenicum album For an itchy, runny nose, sneezing, watery eyes, and symptoms that are better indoors.

Gelsemium For violent bouts of sneezing, a blocked or runny nose, and an itchy throat.

Euphrasia For itchy, watery eyes, especially when the tears feel hot and burn the eyelids. Symptoms are usually better in the evening.

Naturopathy

Increasing your intake of vitamin C and bioflavonoids (a group of compounds found in fruits and vegetables) may help combat allergies—citrus fruits, in particular, are rich sources of both. Pantothenic acid (found in yeast, liver, and eggs) and beta carotene (found in yellow and orange fruits and vegetables) may also relieve the symptoms of allergies.

SINUS PAIN

The sinuses are several air-filled cavities in the bones that surround the nose. Mucus drains through these cavities into narrow ducts, which lead to the nose. Sometimes, however, these ducts become blocked, causing the buildup of mucus in the sinuses. This results in congestion and pain around the upper part of the nose and the forehead. The usual cause of blocked sinuses is a viral infection such as the common cold or influenza.

Another cause of sinus pain is sinusitis (see page 88), which occurs when the membrane lining the sinuses becomes inflamed and infected. Acupressure, reflexology, and hydrotherapy may help alleviate sinus pain.

Acupressure

The acupressure points recommended for allergic rhinitis—Bl 10 and Kid 27—are also thought to help sinus problems.

Reflexology

Reflexologists treat sinus pain by applying sustained pressure to each of the toes. Or you can try a reflexology technique called thumb-walking at home. First, apply a small amount of moisturizing lotion or vegetable oil to the hands and feet. Place the thumb on the foot and gently bend and unbend the thumb at the first joint, moving the pad of the thumb slightly forward as you do so. For sinus pain, thumb-walk the bottom of each toe in turn, starting from the tip down. Do the same on the top of the toes, using your index finger instead of your thumb. Repeat on the opposite foot.

Hydrotherapy

Inhaling steam may help relieve sinus pain. Take long, hot showers or inhale the steam from a bowl of very hot water. Hot, wet compresses placed over the sinuses promote drainage and increase blood flow to the area.

Acupressure for allergic rhinitis

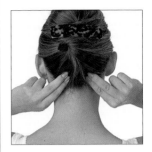

*PRESSURE POINT BL 10
This is found on either side of your spine about two finger widths below the base of your skull.*

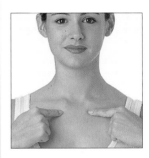

*PRESSURE POINT KID 27
This is located just under your collarbones on either side of your breastbone.*

77

The Hay Fever Sufferer

Pollen allergies are at their worst in early summer. Sufferers experience sneezing, itchy and watery eyes, nasal congestion, and inflammation of the membranes lining the mouth, nose, and throat. In some cases, hay fever can severely disrupt daily life, making it essential to find long-term solutions.

Lucy is 17 and wants to go to college to study veterinary science in the fall. For several years she has suffered from hay fever that lasts from mid-May until late July—and during part of that time she will be taking her final exams. Her symptoms—bouts of sneezing, a runny nose, and itchy, puffy eyes—make it hard for her to concentrate on her studies. Lucy's family lives in a small farming town; she spends a lot of time walking the family dog in local fields and playing outdoor sports. Her parents took her to see the family doctor, who diagnosed an allergy to grass pollen and prescribed antihistamines and a nasal spray. These, however, provide only partial relief, and Lucy wants to find out what other measures she can take.

WHAT LUCY SHOULD DO

Because Lucy knows which allergen is causing her symptoms, she can take some measures to avoid it. When the pollen count is high, she should stay indoors with all of the windows closed; when she needs to go out, wearing sunglasses may help. Lucy can also ask her parents to purchase a particulate air filter, which will dramatically reduce the amount of indoor pollen. She should cut down on dairy products, which are thought to encourage mucus production, and increase her intake of foods that are rich in vitamin C. Because Lucy's symptoms are worse during the day, she could try studying at night. Lucy might also investigate homeopathic remedies for allergies.

Action Plan

DIET
Stop eating cereal with milk for breakfast and cut down on cheese-filled dishes. Instead of drinking coffee with milk, drink lemon or blackcurrant herbal teas. Snack on raw vegetables or citrus fruits.

HEALTH
Get plenty of sleep and minimize the stress of studying by planning schedules carefully.

LIFESTYLE
Stop walking the dog. Play indoor rather than outdoor sports during the summer.

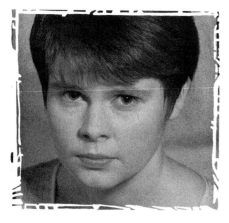

DIET
Eliminating a particular food— dairy products for example—from the diet may alleviate allergy symptoms.

HEALTH
The symptoms of a chronic allergy may in part result from weakened immunity due to stress or to a prior illness.

LIFESTYLE
An adjustment in your daily schedule may be necessary to cope with symptoms.

HOW THINGS TURNED OUT FOR LUCY

With the help and encouragement of her parents—who took over walking the dog, purchased an air filter, and changed their dietary patterns—Lucy put all of the self-help measures into practice. Unfortunately, their impact on her symptoms was not as great as she or her parents hoped. Lucy then went to visit a homeopath and was prescribed a remedy called *Arsenicum album*. She took this regularly and her symptoms became manageable.

THE THROAT

Coughs and sore throats are common symptoms of colds and influenza, but they may also be due to allergies or dry, dusty, or smoky environments that irritate the mucous membranes.

Many throat problems stem from inhaling airborne particles that produce allergic reactions, infections, or irritations. Your tonsils and adenoids, located at the opening of the throat, are there to help protect your upper respiratory tract from infection. Sometimes, however, they are infected by the microorganisms they're intended to fight.

COUGHS

This forceful, sometimes violent, form of respiration helps to expel mucus from the throat or lungs. Coughs are diagnosed by their sounds, by whether they are dry or productive of mucus, and by the color and content of the mucus produced. Characteristic cough sounds include whoops, rattles, barks, and hacks. A productive cough brings forth mucus (sometimes called sputum or phlegm), which is indicative of its cause. Gummy green or yellow mucus indicates an infection; colorless frothy mucus points to an allergic reaction; pink, red, or rust-colored frothy mucus contains blood and is a sign of a ruptured blood vessel in the lungs, nose, or throat.

Smoking, colds (see page 84), influenza (see page 85), bronchitis (see page 98), and passing irritants like dust can all give rise to a cough. It may also be a nervous habit. In some cases, a dry or tickly cough may be relieved by warm, soothing drinks such as honey and water, or throat lozenges, although these tend to be highly sugared. Check with your doctor, however, if your cough is bloody, persistent, severe, or exhausting, because sometimes a cough may have a serious underlying cause, such as lung cancer. Note how long you have had your cough and whether it started suddenly and is worse at certain times, for example, during the night, or after eating or taking exercise. Aromatherapy, herbalism, folk medicine, and homeopathic remedies can help alleviate coughs.

Aromatherapy

Myrrh essential oil may reduce mucus, and frankincense eases difficult breathing (avoid myrrh if you are pregnant). Add either one to a base oil such as sweet almond, and use it to massage the chest and back. Alternatively, put a few drops on a handkerchief and inhale the vapors. Eucalyptus oil can also be used as an inhalant or in a massage.

Herbalism

A mullein infusion may relieve coughs in children and adults; an infusion of white horehound is suitable for adults. An elecampane infusion may help croupy coughs. Aniseed and marsh mallow infusions may relieve unproductive irritating coughs.

Folk medicine

Onions and mustard are traditional cures for chest congestion. Make a cough syrup by placing six chopped onions and ½ cup of honey in a double boiler. Cook slowly for two hours, strain, and take warm as needed. A mustard plaster is made by mixing one part mustard powder with three parts flour and adding enough warm water to make a paste. Spread the paste between two layers of cotton cloth and place on the chest for up to 20 minutes, checking periodically that the mustard does not cause blistering.

Homeopathy

Spongia tosta For dry, harsh coughing.
Bryonia For chest colds and coughing with shallow, painful, panting breathing, pain that is relieved by pressure, and coughs that worsen when you move.
Ipecac For productive, rattling, bronchial coughs, phlegm brought up with difficulty, and coughing that ends with gagging or vomiting. (Take the homeopathic Ipecac, not the identically named over-the-counter drug.)

continued on page 82

STEAM INHALATION
To alleviate a dry, tickly cough, inhale steam from a bowl of very hot water. This will take away the tickle by moistening the mucous membranes of the throat.

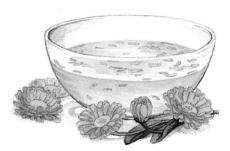

Treating Coughs with

Herbalism

Coughing is a natural mechanism to clear air passages and keep you breathing freely. Rather than trying to suppress a cough, herbalism aims to fight infection, loosen mucus, and soothe and tone the tissues of the respiratory tract.

MARIGOLD INFUSION

If your cough is accompanied by a fever, an infusion of marigold flowers may help to bring your temperature down and increase your immunity. Take 1 table-spoon of the infusion every hour until your temperature is normal.

When you have a cough that is associated with an infection, herbalists believe you need herbs that will build up the immune system and increase your resistance to further complications. They may recommend an infusion made from equal parts of elderflower, peppermint, and yarrow, which not only helps the body fight infection when you are ill but also acts as a preventive. Drink a cup three times a day for six weeks as a preventive measure, and a cup every three hours for two or three

days if you are ill. An infusion made with three parts sage and one part thyme may also be helpful, especially for a bronchial cough that produces thick mucus. If you use fresh herbs, add 2 teaspoons of the herbal mixture to every cup of boiling water; if you use dried herbs, add 1 teaspoon to each cup.

Gargling with an infusion of sage will strengthen the respiratory tract tissue, and make it less prone to infectious illnesses. Avoid sage and thyme during pregnancy.

SOOTHING HERBS

Yarrow, garlic, and rosemary contain active compounds that can help relieve coughs and other associated respiratory tract symptoms. Avoid rosemary during pregnancy.

Yarrow may relieve mucus—drink an infusion of the flowers.

Yarrow tincture can be taken instead of an infusion.

Garlic has antibiotic and expectorant properties—eat plenty of the fresh cloves.

Rosemary in an infusion may relieve coughs associated with chills, colds, and influenza.

Garlic capsules may be taken instead of fresh garlic, although the active ingredient in some brands may be diminished in the processing.

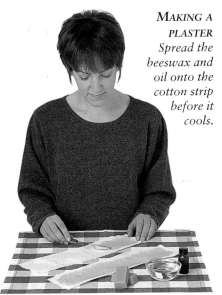

MAKING A PLASTER Spread the beeswax and oil onto the cotton strip before it cools.

HERBAL POULTICES

Poultices and plasters, which are similar to compresses but use the whole herb rather than an infusion, used to be popular home remedies but they have fallen into disuse. They are applied hot and are effective in relieving pain and congestion by improving the blood supply to the area. A cabbage or onion poultice is thought to reduce swelling and inflammation and can be used to treat a cough or throat infection. Dip four large cabbage leaves or onion slices in boiling water to soften them. Pat them dry and place two layers over the throat. Hold in place with a bandage or cotton gauze.

A plaster—a wax-impregnated cloth strip—can also be used to treat a cough and sore throat. Heat 10 drops of an essential oil, such as eucalyptus, thyme, or lemon, with ½ ounce of beeswax and 1 fluid ounce (2 tablepoons) of vegetable oil. Once the wax has melted, remove it from the heat and let the mixture cool until it resembles a creamy paste. Then spread it onto thin strips of cotton cloth. Wrap the strips around the neck or chest; secure with a bandage or cotton gauze. The wax will warm and soften with the body's heat, slowly releasing the essential oil.

HERBS AS INHALANTS

Because central heating dries the air, living or working in a heated environment can dry out your nose and throat. This may give rise to a cough and increase susceptibility to infection. The easiest way to rehydrate the throat is to inhale steam from a cup of herbal tea. Breathe deeply through the nose and mouth alternately, taking the steam down the throat and into the chest. Inhaling the vapors from a chamomile infusion may be therapeutic.

Another way of "inhaling" the aromatic compounds of herbs is to chew a pungent herb like horseradish—this should quickly unblock the sinuses.

A WARMING RUB FOR CHEST INFECTIONS AND COUGHS

Herbalists recommend this rub for relieving a deep rumbling cough that is due to chest and throat infections. To prepare the rub, you need 2 ounces of any of the following dried herbs: peppermint, thyme, rosemary, sage, lemon balm, elecampane, or angelica. You also need 1 teaspoon of ground mustard seed, 1 teaspoon of ground black peppercorns, 1 teaspoon of ground gingerroot, and 16 fluid ounces (2 cups) of vegetable oil.

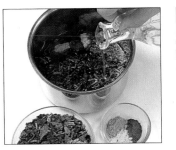

1 *Mix the dried herbs with the mustard, pepper, and ginger. Divide the mixture in half and place half in a small saucepan; cover with the vegetable oil.*

2 *Place the pan in a larger saucepan. Fill the bottom pan with water almost to the top of the small pan. Simmer for two hours.*

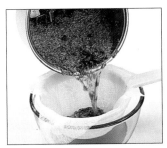

3 *Strain the oil through a sieve. Discard the herbs left in the pan and keep the oil. Pour it over the unused herbs and repeat the process.*

4 *The oil should be rubbed into the chest, throat, and back two to six times daily. It can also be used to make a plaster that can be applied to the chest.*

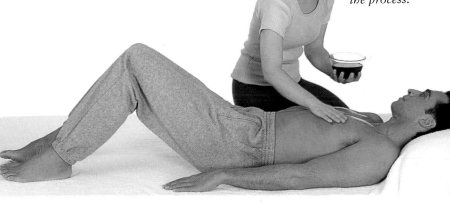

Kali carbonicum For violent spasmodic coughs that are worse in the early hours of the morning and produce copious thick, yellow mucus.

Pulsatilla For a cough that produces thick, yellow-green mucus or a cough that is dry at night and productive during the day.

SORE THROAT

Although there are many causes of a sore throat, it is usually a symptom of a cold (see page 84), influenza (see page 85), or a throat infection (see page 88). Other causes include smoking; being in a dusty, polluted, or a dry, centrally heated environment; having a chronic cough; excessive talking or shouting; or abrasions to the membranes of the throat (from fish bones, for example). Some people find that they wake up with a mild sore throat because they have been breathing through the mouth during the night, causing the mucous membranes of the throat to dry out.

Sore throats vary in severity—from mild discomfort and dryness to acute pain and difficulty swallowing. The latter usually signals a throat infection. See a doctor if it is painful to swallow, if you have a high fever, or if a severe sore throat does not clear up within three to four days.

The treatment for sore throat depends on the cause. An immediate home remedy for the characteristic tickling or rawness of a sore throat is a warm saltwater gargle. The hotter the water the better, but be careful not to scald your mouth. Use only mildly warm water when administering a saltwater gargle to children. Aspirin or acetaminophen will relieve pain (do not give aspirin to children). The conventional treatment for a bacterial throat infection is an antibiotic.

Inhaling the vapors of, or applying rubs made from, essential oils, drinking herbal infusions, or taking a homeopathic remedy may help alleviate a mild sore throat.

Aromatherapy

Steam inhalations of lavender, thyme, or eucalyptus essential oils can be soothing (avoid thyme during pregnancy). A gargle made from one drop each of oil of lemon and sandalwood in a glass of water may be taken up to three times a day.

A rub made from eucalyptus and peppermint oil added to a base oil can be applied to the chest and throat. This is particularly soothing if the tonsils are inflamed. Seek advice from an aromatherapist before applying such rubs to children's skin.

Herbalism

The natural mucilage—gummy substance—in marsh mallow and slippery elm bark helps ease sore throats when taken as an infusion. Sage infusion makes a soothing gargle, which can be used twice a day, or every hour if your throat is very inflamed. If your sore throat is caused by a mouth or gum infection, add myrrh to the gargle; this will reduce irritation. (Avoid sage and myrrh during pregnancy.) Gargle with an infusion of calendula or the tincture diluted with warm water. If you find herbal infusions unpalatable, sweeten them with honey; this will also help to soothe inflammation.

Both garlic and onions are good antiseptics and decongestants, and garlic has antibiotic qualities. Garlic and onions can be prepared in various ways—you can eat them raw or roasted, or you can even drink them boiled in milk.

Homeopathy

Belladonna For sore throats with a sudden onset, fever, and flushed skin.

Hepar sulphuris For a severe sore throat with pus formation, pain that shoots to your ears when you swallow, or the sensation of something stuck in your throat.

Phytolacca For a throat that is so sore that you cannot swallow.

Lycopodium For soreness concentrated on the right side of the throat, or starting there and moving left.

Lachesis For left-sided pain or pain that starts there and moves right.

SORE THROAT AND SMOKING

Smokers often suffer from a persistent sore throat because inhaling tobacco smoke irritates the larynx and the mucous membranes that line the throat. Heavy smoking can also cause chronic bronchitis, which gives rise to the characteristic "smoker's cough"; a sore throat may be a secondary symptom of this. The only way to eliminate this chronic sore throat is to stop smoking. Occasionally, a sore throat associated with smoking is a sign of pharyngeal cancer.

CHAPTER 6

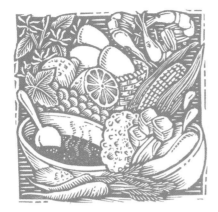

ILLNESSES AND INFECTIONS

*Conventional medicine treats infections
with antibiotics, antifungals, and drugs to
alleviate symptoms. Although antibiotics are a
powerful weapon, they may also destroy the body's
friendly bacteria, allowing fungal infections to
flourish. They may also interfere with the efficacy
of other drugs like the oral contraceptive pill.
Therapies such as homeopathy and herbalism
offer a gentler form of treatment.*

COMMON INFECTIONS

When your body's immune system is weakened, you become more vulnerable to common infections. Natural remedies can help ease discomfort and strengthen your resistance.

Common infections eventually affect everyone. They are usually short-lived and include illnesses like colds and flu, and throat, sinus, eye, and urinary tract infections. Infections may be bacterial or viral and they often enter the body through inhaled droplets of liquid that have been sneezed or coughed into the air.

THE COMMON COLD

There are nearly 200 cold viruses that cause the mucous membranes lining the nose and throat to become inflamed, resulting in a runny, stuffy nose (see page 76) and a sore throat (see page 82). Other symptoms include headache, chills, slight fever, aches and pains, and fatigue. Most colds clear up within a few days, but recurrent colds may be a sign that you are run-down, possibly due to poor diet, stress, or illness.

Many painkillers, decongestants, and antihistamines are available over the counter for temporary relief from cold symptoms, but there is no drug that can cure the common cold. The following natural remedies may help relieve your symptoms or lessen your chances of catching a cold in the first place.

Homeopathy

Aconite For the first signs of a cold, such as sneezing and a burning throat.
Belladonna For colds with a high temperature, a sore throat, and a tickly cough.
Ferrum phosphate For colds that start slowly with a mild fever.
Gelsemium For flulike colds accompanied by shivering, chills, aching, and heaviness.
Euphrasia For streaming eyes and nose.

Herbalism

Infusions of cinnamon, angelica, or ginger are good for chills; peppermint and yarrow help reduce fever and promote sweating; elderflower may reduce mucus; and marsh mallow is an expectorant. For recurrent colds, echinacea tincture or capsules and an infusion of goldenseal may boost the immune system (avoid goldenseal if you are pregnant or have hypertension).

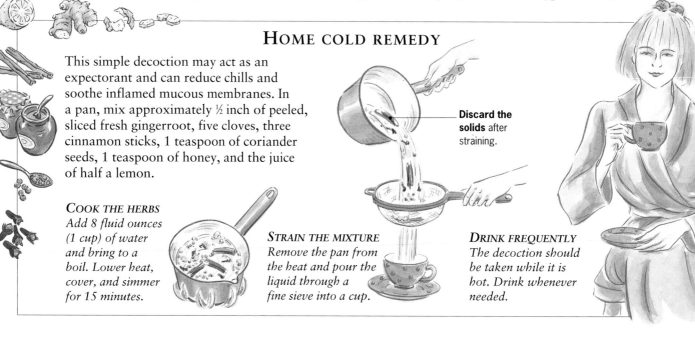

HOME COLD REMEDY

This simple decoction may act as an expectorant and can reduce chills and soothe inflamed mucous membranes. In a pan, mix approximately ½ inch of peeled, sliced fresh gingerroot, five cloves, three cinnamon sticks, 1 teaspoon of coriander seeds, 1 teaspoon of honey, and the juice of half a lemon.

Discard the solids after straining.

COOK THE HERBS
Add 8 fluid ounces (1 cup) of water and bring to a boil. Lower heat, cover, and simmer for 15 minutes.

STRAIN THE MIXTURE
Remove the pan from the heat and pour the liquid through a fine sieve into a cup.

DRINK FREQUENTLY
The decoction should be taken while it is hot. Drink whenever needed.

Chinese herbalism

Colds are thought to be caused by the invasion of Wind-Cold. To eliminate this, an herbalist may recommend a standard decoction called Cong Chi Tang. This consists of Cong Bai (the heads of green onions) and Dan Dou Chi (soy beans) simmered in water for 15 minutes, then strained.

Acupressure

Apply pressure to GV 14 and Lu 7 to alleviate cold symptoms, and to LI 4 (see page 68), which is found on the webbed area between the thumb and first finger, to boost the body's energy (avoid LI 4 during pregnancy).

Hydrotherapy

Cold friction rubs are thought to boost immunity: sufferers are warmed in a hot bath or steam room, briskly rubbed with a cold, wet cloth, then wrapped in a blanket. Daily alternating hot and cold showers are also recommended to prevent colds.

If you already have a cold, make a foot bath with 1 tablespoon of dried mustard to 2 pints of hot water.

Naturopathy

Large doses of vitamin C are advocated for preventing colds—if there is a cold outbreak, take at least 1,000 milligrams a day. Vitamin A (found in liver) and zinc (found in shellfish) are also thought to strengthen the body's immune system.

INFLUENZA

A viral infection of the respiratory tract, influenza, or flu, causes aches, fatigue, chills and fever, sweating, loss of appetite, and a general feeling of ill health. Sometimes flu is accompanied by nausea. These symptoms are often followed by a cough (see page 79), sore throat (see page 82), and nasal congestion (see page 76). The fever and other symptoms subside after about two days. Generally, symptoms disappear completely within five days, although respiratory symptoms and weakness may last longer.

Although there are outbreaks of influenza each winter, an epidemic of major proportions occurs only every few years. People most susceptible to flu have weakened immune systems at the time of exposure to the virus, so general good health offers the best protection.

Flu vaccinations also help prevent infection, but they are effective for only 60 to 70 percent of those vaccinated, and they must be repeated every year.

Conventional treatment for flu is bed rest and a painkiller such as aspirin or acetaminophen. (Do not give aspirin to children.) Occasionally, flu can develop into a serious illness such as pneumonia, in which case antiviral drugs may be prescribed.

Homeopathy, Western and Eastern herbalism, and acupressure may alleviate flu symptoms and help fight infection.

Homeopathy

Aconite For flu symptoms accompanied by anxiety, agitation, and thirst.

Ferrum phosphate For the gradual onset of mild fever and sweating.

Belladonna For sudden, very high fever and a throbbing headache.

Gelsemium For chills up and down the spine, fatigue, weakness, shaking, and a throbbing headache.

Arsenicum album For exhaustion and streaming eyes and nose.

Eupatorium For severe pains in the limbs and a splitting headache.

Herbalism

A peppermint infusion may be useful for nausea, elderflower may ease sore throats, boneset is advised for aching muscles, and vervain may encourage sweating and reduce fever (avoid vervain during pregnancy). A

continued on page 88

Acupressure points for colds

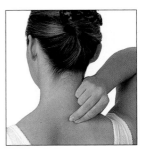

PRESSURE POINT GV 14
This is just below the prominent vertebra at the base of the neck.

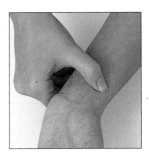

PRESSURE POINT LU 7
This is one finger width above the wrist crease on the line of the pulse.

SYMPTOMS OF INFLUENZA
General flu symptoms manifest themselves in the upper part of the respiratory system, although there can be overall muscle weakness, aching joints, and loss of appetite.

Headaches and fever.

Congested or runny nose.

Cough and sore throat.

Muscle weakness and aching joints.

Shivering attacks alternating with sweating.

Loss of appetite.

Exercise

Regular exercise can help protect you from common and serious disorders. In fact, it is one of the most effective ways of boosting your immune system. Even when you are ill, gentle exercise can make a tremendous difference in the way you feel.

HOW TO EXERCISE SAFELY

Whether you jog, swim, walk, cycle, or do aerobics, you should warm up properly and follow these guidelines.

▶ *Do not eat for two hours before exercising.*

▶ *Wear loose-fitting cotton clothes.*

▶ *Start exercising slowly and build up your endurance over a period of two or three weeks.*

▶ *Take regular sips of water to replace the fluid lost in sweat.*

▶ *Cool down after exercising by gradually slowing the pace of your workout for 5 to 10 minutes.*

Exercise not only makes the body better able to resist infections it also causes the release of endorphins and enkephalins—pain-blocking substances produced by certain cells in the body.

Any exercise that increases the heart and breathing rates is called aerobic. In order to improve your cardiovascular and respiratory fitness, you need to engage in aerobic exercise for at least 20 minutes, three times every week. To warm up before an aerobic workout, gently stretch your muscles using the movements on these pages.

To cool down after aerobic exercise, reverse the order of movements slowly so that your heart rate and breathing gradually return to normal. This will prevent the buildup of lactic acid in the muscles.

Illness is no reason for not exercising—in fact, light exercise can often significantly improve your sense of well-being and promote recovery. If you have a minor infection such as a cold, going for a walk, doing stretching exercises, deep breathing, or yoga may bring relief. Avoid anything more vigorous because this can make your symptoms worse.

Even if you are confined to bed, you can still exercise your muscles by lifting your limbs and your head. You can also use resistance—flex your muscles by pushing or pulling against a bed or wall.

WARMING UP

Whatever form of exercise you choose, the routine illustrated here will prepare your muscles so that you do not damage them. This stretch routine also increases your overall flexibility and it can be used during the day as an energizing break from prolonged standing or sitting.

Spend 5 to 10 minutes warming up. Ease into stretches, gradually extending the stretch as the muscle relaxes and lengthens. Avoid jerky or bouncing movements, and, if you feel any pain, stop immediately.

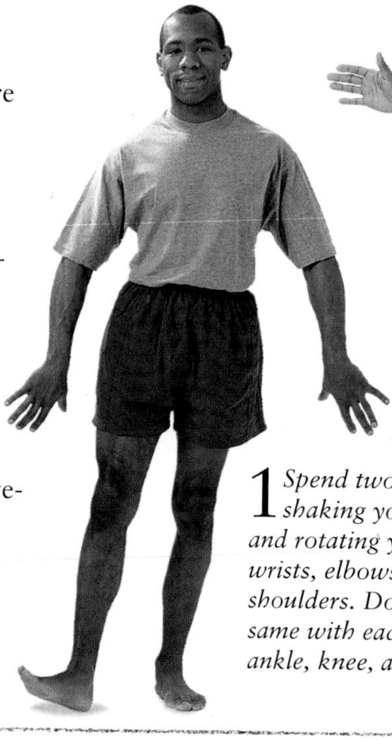

1 *Spend two minutes shaking your hands and rotating your wrists, elbows, and shoulders. Do the same with each ankle, knee, and hip.*

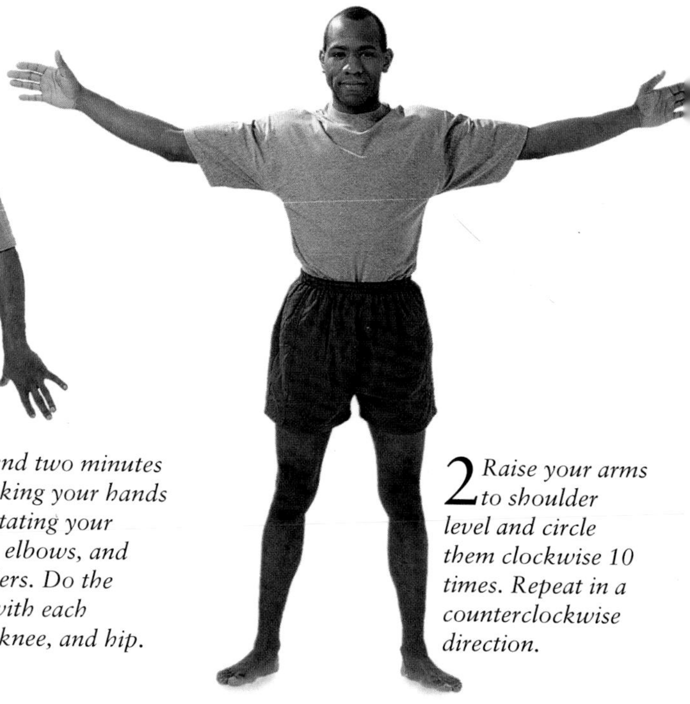

2 *Raise your arms to shoulder level and circle them clockwise 10 times. Repeat in a counterclockwise direction.*

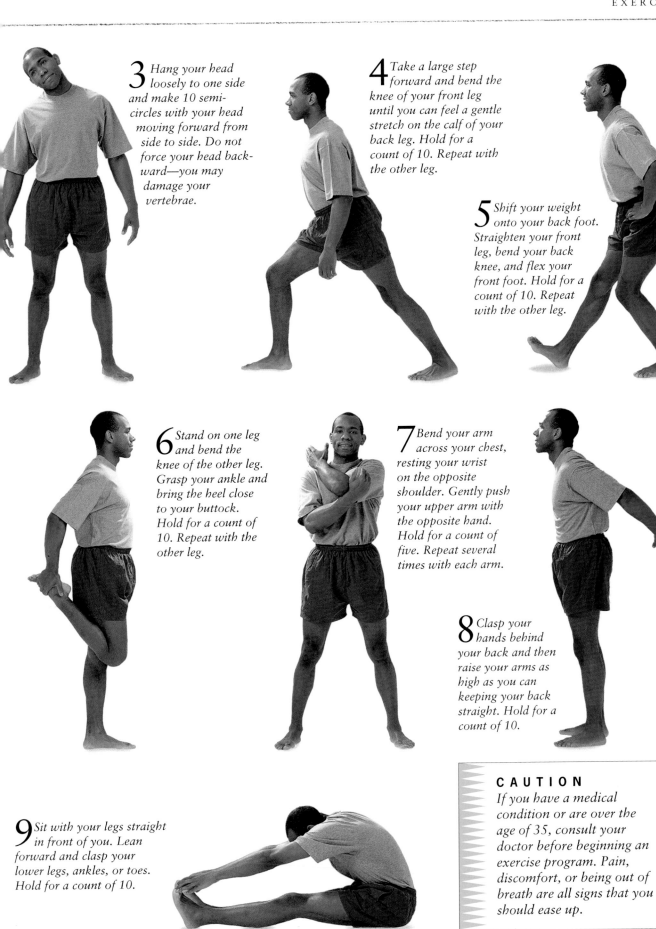

3 Hang your head loosely to one side and make 10 semicircles with your head moving forward from side to side. Do not force your head backward—you may damage your vertebrae.

4 Take a large step forward and bend the knee of your front leg until you can feel a gentle stretch on the calf of your back leg. Hold for a count of 10. Repeat with the other leg.

5 Shift your weight onto your back foot. Straighten your front leg, bend your back knee, and flex your front foot. Hold for a count of 10. Repeat with the other leg.

6 Stand on one leg and bend the knee of the other leg. Grasp your ankle and bring the heel close to your buttock. Hold for a count of 10. Repeat with the other leg.

7 Bend your arm across your chest, resting your wrist on the opposite shoulder. Gently push your upper arm with the opposite hand. Hold for a count of five. Repeat several times with each arm.

8 Clasp your hands behind your back and then raise your arms as high as you can keeping your back straight. Hold for a count of 10.

9 Sit with your legs straight in front of you. Lean forward and clasp your lower legs, ankles, or toes. Hold for a count of 10.

CAUTION
If you have a medical condition or are over the age of 35, consult your doctor before beginning an exercise program. Pain, discomfort, or being out of breath are all signs that you should ease up.

Acupressure for influenza

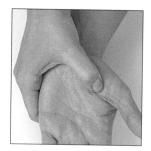

PRESSURE POINT LU 10
This is found two finger widths down from the wrist crease, along the palm side of the thumb.

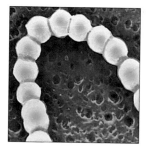

STREPTOCOCCI
Many sore throats and fevers are caused by the streptococcus bacterium (hence "strep throat"), although in some people it causes no symptoms. Streptococci are spherical bacteria that typically form chains.

KEEPING UP YOUR FLUID INTAKE
To lubricate the throat and speed recovery, drink fruit juice, herbal teas, and vegetable soups.

lavender compress may help ease feverish headaches. Taking general tonic herbs, such as echinacea, ginseng, and garlic to boost the immune system may also be helpful (avoid ginseng if you suffer from hypertension).

Chinese herbalism
In China, flu is believed to be due to Wind-Heat invasion. A widely used remedy to clear Wind-Heat is Yin Chiao San (lonicera and forsythia powder), available in pill form. It is thought to relieve symptoms and rid the body of the flu virus if pills are taken as soon as the symptoms start and for up to three days afterward.

Acupressure
To alleviate flu symptoms, apply pressure to either LI 11 (see page 37), which is at the end of the outside elbow crease, or Lu 10.

THROAT INFECTION
Although a mild sore throat (see page 82) may be due to smoking or being in a smoky or dry, centrally heated environment, the usual cause is a viral or bacterial infection. The parts of the throat that usually become infected are the tonsils, larynx, and pharynx. Infections may be accompanied by fever, and swallowing may be difficult. Sometimes, serious illnesses such as cancer may produce hoarseness or a sore throat, so see your doctor if symptoms persist.

There is no cure for a viral throat infection, but if you have a bacterial throat infection, such as strep throat, your doctor may prescribe an antibiotic. Gargling with salt water and taking aspirin may bring pain relief. (Children should be given acetaminophen, not aspirin).

Herbalism and naturopathy may help relieve symptoms or strengthen the body's resistance to infection.

Herbalism
Thyme's antibacterial and antiviral properties may help throat infections. An old folk remedy is to chew fresh sprigs of thyme several times a day.

Elderflower and myrrh may be useful for their decongestant properties, plantain for its ability to soothe mucous membranes, and sage for its antibacterial and antiseptic properties. Rosemary can be taken to alleviate the symptoms of colds and flu that accompany a throat infection. Take all these herbs as infusions. Do not take thyme, myrrh, sage, or rosemary during pregnancy.

Naturopathy
Zinc and vitamins A and C are among the most important nutrients that help fight infection. To obtain them, try to eat at least five servings of fruits and vegetables a day and include plenty of eggs, poultry, and seafood in your diet.

Garlic, with its antibacterial properties, may be helpful, and cabbage and onions also have useful antibacterial properties. Drink lots of fluids such as fruit juices, herbal teas, and vegetable broths. Avoid refined sugars, red meat, white flour, and caffeine.

SINUSITIS
Some of your facial bones contain cavities lined with mucous membranes. Any condition that produces mucus—an allergy or a viral or bacterial infection, for example—can inflame the membranes in the sinuses, causing congestion and pain (see page 77). If the membranes then become infected with bacteria, you have sinusitis. Some people are very susceptible to sinusitis and find that they have an attack every time they catch a common cold.

Although sinusitis is usually a complication of a viral infection, it also may be caused by nasal polyps (growths on the mucous membranes inside the nose), tumors, or physical abnormalities that inhibit sinus drainage. Facial injuries, inhaling infected water (by swimming in a lake, for example), or an abscess on an upper tooth are other less common causes of sinusitis.

The main symptoms of sinusitis are a stuffy, runny nose and a feeling of congestion and pain around the sinus area. You may also have a headache, an earache, and a postnasal drip (a watery or sticky discharge from the back of the nose into the throat). Loss of smell is common and you may have a fever. If your symptoms are persistent or recurrent, see your doctor. Sinusitis is more serious than blocked sinuses and it needs to be treated with antibiotics. A doctor may also prescribe a decongestant nasal spray. In

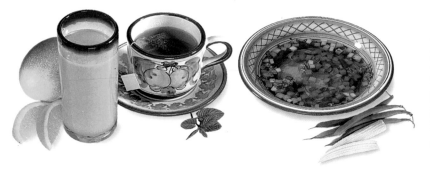

cases that do not respond to treatment, surgical drainage of the affected sinuses may be recommended.

Hydrotherapy and homeopathy may help to alleviate symptoms and eliminate the underlying infection.

Hydrotherapy
An old remedy for sinus problems is rinsing the sinuses with warm salt water. Dissolve ⅛ to ¼ teaspoon of salt (preferably sea salt or kosher salt, which contain fewer impurities than ordinary table salt) in a cup of tepid water. Inhale the water (or squirt it with an eyedropper) into one nostril and tip your head sideways so that the liquid passes across the septum. Let the water run out of the other nostril and then blow your nose. Repeat with the other nostril. Steam inhalations may also be helpful.

Another hydrotherapy technique that may provide symptom relief is the alternate application of hot and cold water. Start by splashing your face with hot water for two minutes, then splash with cold water for one minute. Keep alternating between hot and cold water for 10 to 15 minutes.

Homeopathy
Kali bichromicum For pain in the cheekbones or pressure on the bridge of the nose.
Mercurius solubilis For severe facial pain that gets worse in the cold.
Hepar sulphuris For pain that is concentrated at the back of the nose and is made worse by simple head or eye movements.
Pulsatilla For sinus pain that is accompanied by nausea or indigestion.

CONJUNCTIVITIS
When the membranes lining the eyelid and eyeball—the conjunctiva—become infected or suffer an allergic reaction, they become inflamed. The eye feels itchy and gritty, and there may be a sticky yellow discharge. In allergic conjunctivitis, the discharge is clear—indicating an absence of infection—and the eyelids are swollen and red.

Most conjunctivitis infections are caused by bacteria spread by hand-to-eye contact, or viruses associated with colds, influenza, and sore throats. To avoid spreading the infection or reinfecting yourself, wash your hands often and use disposable paper towels.

Eyedrops or ointment containing antibiotics are prescribed for infections, antihistamines for allergies. Viral conditions usually improve without treatment. Hydrotherapy, homeopathy, and herbalism may help relieve or clear up conjunctivitis. Consult your doctor if symptoms are no better in 24 hours.

Homeopathy
Aconite For conjunctivitis, especially after exposure to cold winds.

HERBAL REMEDIES FOR FEVER

A fever is a symptom of many common infections. It is medically defined as a body temperature of over 98.6°F, taken orally. Depending on the illness, fever may be accompanied by other symptoms such as chills, headache, sweating, thirst, flushed skin, rapid breathing, confusion, or, in severe cases, convulsions. If you have a very high fever or a fever that lasts for more than three days, see your doctor.

Infusions of peppermint, elderflower, yarrow, limeflower, or meadowsweet are recommended by herbalists to reduce fever (avoid meadowsweet during pregnancy). A boneset infusion may help relieve aching muscles, and a lavender compress is cooling. If you have chills as well as fever, try taking decoctions of warming herbs like ginger or cinnamon (see page 84).

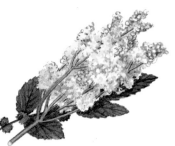

MEADOWSWEET
This is an herb that contains salicylates—substances similar to those in aspirin. An infusion of meadowsweet is anti-inflammatory and promotes sweating.

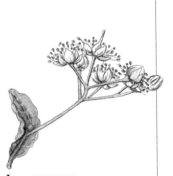

LIMEFLOWER
An infusion of the flowers of lime trees can help to induce sweating, which will lower body temperature.

Hydrotherapy

Water treatments are effective in reducing a high fever quickly. Sponging the body with tepid water, wet packs, and cold compresses are easy self-help measures that will make you feel more comfortable and are easy to practice at home.

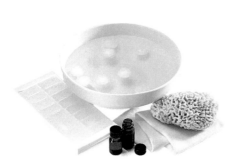

THE COOLING EFFECTS OF WATER
A cold compress is a fast, effective way to reduce the temperature of the body during a fever. Sponging down the body with tepid water can also help.

If your temperature is over 102°F, sponging with water may help bring it down. Tepid rather than cold water should be used because cold water will cause the blood vessels all over the body to constrict—a mechanism that preserves body heat.

Alternatively, try applying a wet pack. Take a towel, soak it in tepid water, apply it to the chest or abdomen, and cover the body with a dry blanket. Leave the pack in place for up to three hours.

Many people believe that a cold bath will reduce a fever, but although this can be effective, it can also exacerbate a fever and should be supervised by a health care professional. What you can do safely is to soak in a tepid bath with ½ pound of Epsom salts or a few drops of sage oil added to help induce sweating. (Avoid sage if pregnant.)

When you have a fever you may lose a lot of fluid through sweating. To prevent dehydration, drink 8 pints of water a day.

COLD COMPRESSES AND TEPID SPONGING

To help cool the body and make a feverish person feel better, apply wet compresses or sponges to the body.

A cold compress has a local effect on the forehead; sponging will make the whole body cool. Tepid water should be used for sponging so that the body does not overheat.

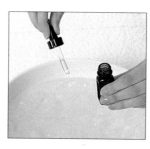

ADD ESSENTIAL OIL
Five drops of lavender oil added to a bowl of ice cold water will help fever accompanied by headache.

SOAK THE COMPRESS
Fold some absorbent fabric into a rectangle and dip in the bowl of water. Wring out the excess water.

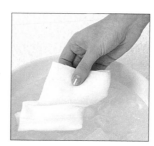

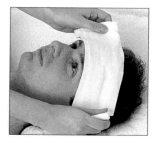

APPLY THE COMPRESS
Place the cold compress on the forehead. Replace as soon as it becomes warm.

TEPID SPONGING
Soak a sponge or washcloth in tepid water, squeeze out, and use to bathe the entire body. Check the patient's temperature frequently. When it is reduced, cover the whole body with a sheet or light blanket.

A sea sponge is absorbent and soft on the skin.

Place a large towel underneath the patient.

Argentum nitrate For copious discharge from the eye.

Pulsatilla For profuse, thick, yellow-green discharge from the eye.

Naturopathy

Practitioners make up a poultice of grated apple or grated raw red-skinned potato, which they place over the (closed) eye once a day for about half an hour. This should reduce eyelid swelling and clear up simple conjunctivitis within two or three days.

Hydrotherapy

To wipe away the discharge, use cotton dipped in warm sterile water—a separate piece of cotton for each eye. To promote healing, apply a compress of gauze dipped in saline solution made with 1 teaspoon of salt and 8 fluid ounces (1 cup) boiled water. Or rinse daily with a milder solution—1 teaspoon salt in 16 fluid ounces (2 cups) water.

URINARY TRACT INFECTIONS

Infections can affect any part of the urinary tract from the urethra (urethritis) to the kidneys (pyelonephritis), but one of the most common urinary tract infections is cystitis, which is an inflammation of the bladder. Cystitis is more common in women than men because women have a shorter urethra and so bacteria have a shorter distance to travel to infect the bladder.

The symptoms of cystitis include the urgent, frequent desire to urinate, leaking urine involuntarily, burning or pain on urination, and blood in the urine. An infection of the kidney and ureters should be suspected if there is pain in the back and lower abdomen, nausea, fever, and lethargy.

Cystitis in women may be caused by bacteria passing from the anus to the urethra due to poor hygiene after a bowel movement. Other causes include bruising during intercourse, irritation to the bladder from highly perfumed toiletries, or wearing tight pants or synthetic underwear.

You can avoid urinary tract infections by drinking plenty of fluids (preferably water), emptying the bladder regularly (particularly after sexual intercourse), and taking care with personal hygiene. Wear cotton underwear and loose-fitting pants.

One teaspoon of sodium bicarbonate taken in a glass of water can help relieve the symptoms of cystitis. Take once every three hours. Most urinary tract infections are treated with antibiotics. Naturopathy, herbalism, aromatherapy, and homeopathy can help relieve discomfort.

Naturopathy

Drink two or three glasses of water at the first sign of an attack and then drink a glass of bland liquid, such as herbal tea, every 20 minutes. Drinking cranberry juice regularly can prevent some urinary tract infections because it contains compounds that are thought to prevent bacteria from attaching themselves to the walls of the bladder.

Avoid salt, red meat, spicy foods, greasy foods, alcohol, and caffeine during an attack, or give them up entirely if you suffer from chronic infections.

Herbalism

An infusion of plantain and thyme is advised at the beginning of a urinary tract infection. During an attack try buchu leaves in an infusion—they may act as a diuretic and urinary antiseptic. (Avoid thyme and buchu leaves during pregnancy or while breast feeding.) Infusions of couch grass, marsh mallow, nettle, and yarrow may soothe the urinary tract.

Aromatherapy

Add two drops each of juniper berry, eucalyptus, and sandalwood essential oils to a warm bath or, alternatively, six drops of bergamot. Hot compresses made with chamomile and tea tree essential oils may help ease pain when applied to the lower part of the abdomen.

Homeopathy

Nux vomica For the frequent urge to urinate and painful urination.

Cantharis For burning, cutting pains in the lower abdomen, the nonstop urge to urinate, and a dull ache in the lower back.

Apis mel For sharp stinging pains in the lower abdomen and scanty hot urine.

Belladonna For pain and burning sensations in the urethra and bladder, and sensitivity to movement.

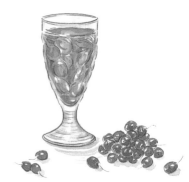

CRANBERRY JUICE
Cranberry juice contains compounds that may help prevent urinary tract infections, such as cystitis. Chronic sufferers should drink two to four glasses of cranberry juice daily.

A Chronic Cystitis Sufferer

Cystitis, an inflammation of the bladder, is usually caused by bacteria and often is brought on by poor hygiene, stress, an unhealthy diet, tight clothing, or sexual intercourse. The two main symptoms are a persistent need to urinate and pain on passing urine. In cases of chronic cystitis, you must discover the cause of the infection to prevent recurring attacks.

Sarah is a 35-year-old working mother. She has two children—an eight-year-old son and a five-year-old daughter. She returned to full-time work as a teacher when her daughter began school six months ago. Her husband, James, has a busy, stressful job as a computer systems analyst. Pressures at work and at home have created tension between Sarah and James, and the arguments have made communication difficult.

For the past few months, Sarah has suffered from a heavy, dull, aching sensation in her lower pelvis, and sudden urges to urinate, but when she gets to the toilet she passes almost no urine and she has acute burning pains in her bladder.

When the problem first started, Sarah treated herself with sodium bicarbonate powder, which she bought over the counter at a drugstore. It helped slightly, but Sarah decided to see her doctor when she still had symptoms two days later.

The doctor told her that she probably had cystitis—a bladder infection—and he prescribed a course of antibiotics, took a urine sample, and told her to return for further consultation if the antibiotics didn't help.

Sarah took the full course of antibiotics as directed and her symptoms eased. A few months later, however, the symptoms recurred. Sarah returned to her doctor, who suggested that Sarah assess her diet and lifestyle and pay attention to personal hygiene, particularly after bowel movements and sexual intercourse, if she was going to prevent frequent recurrences of the cystitis.

Sarah admitted that she had been under pressure at home and work, and decided to think carefully about the possible causes of her symptoms.

PERSONAL HYGIENE
Bacteria from the anus are easily transferred to the urethra and the bladder. It is important to wipe from the front to the back after a bowel movement. Perfumed toiletries can irritate the opening to the urethra.

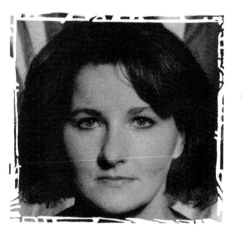

SEX LIFE
Failing to empty the bladder after sex, or using scented creams for lubrication or a diaphragm for contraception can cause cystitis. Sometimes, vigorous sex can irritate the urethra, thus making it susceptible to infection.

DIET
Not enough fluids and a diet high in fat, red meat, dairy products, pickles, coffee, alcohol, sugar, and salt can irritate the bladder.

CLOTHES
Wearing nylon underwear, tights, or tight pants, can provide a perfect environment for bacteria. Some detergents aggravate cystitis.

LIFESTYLE
A busy, stressful life with not enough time to rest or eat properly can undermine your natural immunity and lead to chronic infections such as cystitis.

WHAT SARAH SHOULD DO

Sarah should drink plenty of fluids—at least 5 pints a day; urinate regularly (always after sex); and pay careful attention to her personal and sexual hygiene. Washing thoroughly with water and three drops of witch hazel solution after sex may be helpful. Sarah's husband, James, should wash his genitals and rinse away any soap before sex.

Herbal infusions made from yarrow, marsh mallow, couch grass, or nettle can encourage urination and soothe the bladder and urethra.

Sarah should replace all of her synthetic underwear with loose-fitting cotton panties, which will allow air to circulate and her skin to breathe. She should also avoid tight-fitting pants and tights.

Foods that may help alleviate cystitis include barley and barley water, cranberries, pumpkin seeds, dandelion, aduki beans, and onions. Sarah should avoid dairy products, sugar, salt, citrus fruits, pickles, vinegar, rhubarb, strawberries, coffee, processed foods, and alcohol.

Because her daughter has recently started school and Sarah has just returned to work, she is under a lot more stress than usual. She needs to compensate for this with rest and relaxation. She also needs to discuss her problems fully with her husband. She must try to make James see that she is not angry with him but that she needs more support.

Action Plan

LIFESTYLE
Discuss with James ways to lighten the load of domestic responsibilities. Think about getting help at home. Try to spend more time alone with James. Spend more time relaxing. Take up yoga.

DIET
Cut down on sugar and caffeine. Drink plenty of fluids including herbal teas and cranberry juice. Eat a healthy balanced diet, with plenty of fresh fruit, vegetables, and whole grains. Cut down on citrus fruits, red meat, and dairy products.

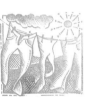

PERSONAL HYGIENE
Stop using perfumed products such as bubble bath. Replace usual soap with unperfumed soap. Practice good hygiene after a bowel movement and wash if possible.

CLOTHES
Don't wear synthetic underwear and tights. Choose cotton panties, and tights with a cotton gusset. Make sure that all clothes, particularly underwear, are thoroughly rinsed after washing.

SEX LIFE
Make sure that James is conscientiously hygienic. Empty the bladder and wash after sexual intercourse. Try some new positions if familiar ones are painful. If using a diaphragm, make sure it fits properly, or switch to another method of birth control.

HOW THINGS TURNED OUT FOR SARAH

Sarah adopted self-help measures such as drinking plenty of water and being scrupulous about her personal and sexual hygiene, but she did not eliminate caffeine from her diet. She found that her symptoms abated, only to return when she was feeling particularly stressed or tired.

Although she discussed the burden of domestic responsibilities with her husband and they hired a cleaning service, Sarah still felt that all of her time was taken up with work and caring for her children.

Sarah decided to seek help from a homeopath. She was prescribed a constitutional remedy, one that treats the overall state of the body. Since taking the remedy, Sarah has become interested in other natural remedies. She has started a yoga class and she is adapting her diet to include more nutritious foods. She is aware that if she allows herself to become stressed and she neglects her self-help techniques the cystitis will recur. For the moment, however, she feels in control.

Through yoga, Sarah has learned to relax and focus her mind and body. She has found that even half an hour of relaxation helps her feel more confident about the pressures in her life, and less overwhelmed about the demands that her husband and children, her job, and her home make on her time. She feels she has more time for herself.

INFECTIOUS DISEASES

Children are afflicted by a number of highly contagious diseases that also affect unprotected adults. Natural remedies can help ease their symptoms.

Whereas common infections such as colds and flu can attack repeatedly, one bout with measles or mumps may confer lifelong immunity. The latter diseases usually affect children, but older people and young adults may also fall victim. Many of these illnesses can be avoided with immunization at an early age—all should be treated with conventional medicine before natural therapies.

MONONUCLEOSIS

Infectious mononucleosis, or glandular fever, is a viral infection characterized by a severe sore throat (tonsillitis), swollen glands—particularly around the neck, armpits, and groin—headache, high fever, and general ill health. Sometimes the liver and spleen are mildly affected, and fatigue and depression occur. The only conventional treatments for mononucleosis are bed rest and analgesics to relieve pain and fever. Most people recover within six weeks but often feel depressed and lethargic for two to three months after other symptoms have gone.

Because mononucleosis is a long and debilitating infection, natural remedies, such as homeopathy, Chinese herbalism, and naturopathy, are useful for boosting the body's immune system and natural healing

powers. Bach flower remedies may alleviate the symptoms of emotional debility.

Homeopathy
Belladonna For the sudden onset of symptoms, high fever, and a red face.
Baryta carbonica For swollen glands.
Calcarea phosphorica For swollen glands and debility after acute disease.
Mercurius solubilis For excessive perspiration, tonsillitis, tender glands, and symptoms that become worse at night.

Chinese herbalism
Common features of mononucleosis are thought to be Heat in the Blood, Liver, and Stomach; and deficiencies of Energy, Yin, and sometimes Blood. Herbs such as Chi Shao Yao (red peony root), Jin Yin Hua (honeysuckle flowers), Lian Qiao (forsythia fruit), Ju Hua (chrysanthemum flowers), and Pu Gong Ying (dandelion) are used to eliminate Heat from the body. For an Energy deficiency, a Chinese herbalist may give a tonic prescription such as Yu Ping Feng San (jade screen powder).

Naturopathy
Eat a balanced diet with plenty of fresh fruits and vegetables, fruit juices, vegetable soups, whole grains, eggs, seeds, nuts, fish, and liver. Fresh fruits and vegetables in particular are rich in healing vitamins and minerals. It is a good idea to eat fresh garlic, or include extra garlic in cooking, and to drink plenty of water.

Avoid red meat, spicy foods, fatty foods, dairy products, processed foods, additives, caffeine, and alcohol.

Bach flower remedies
Try olive for feelings of fatigue, sweet chestnut for dejection or depression, and oak if you feel unable to cope with illness. You can use a combination of Bach flower remedies in order to suit your particular needs and symptoms. Put a few drops of the remedy in a beverage, or place directly under the tongue.

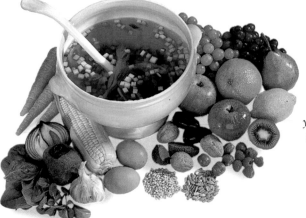

FOODS FOR CONVALESCENCE Although your appetite may be diminished after a debilitating illness, you must keep up your intake of vitamins and minerals. Eat easily digested foods such as soups, steamed vegetables, and fruit.

CHICKENPOX

Caused by the varicella-zoster virus, chickenpox is a common infectious disease of childhood that is spread in airborne droplets Symptoms appear two to three weeks after infection and include an itchy rash and a mild fever. Occasionally, adult sufferers develop pneumonia, but fortunately most people have chickenpox before the age of 10, when it generally runs its course without complications. Although a bout of chickenpox provides lifelong immunity, the virus remains dormant in certain nerve tissues and may reappear later in life in the form of shingles (herpes zoster).

Conventional treatment for chickenpox is bed rest and aspirin or acetaminophen (do not give aspirin to children) to reduce fever and calamine lotion to relieve itching.

Therapies such as hydrotherapy, aromatherapy, and Chinese herbalism may relieve the symptoms of chickenpox.

Hydrotherapy

Applying cool, wet towels to the rash can relieve itchiness. Soaking in a lukewarm bath with finely ground oatmeal or baking soda added may be helpful, particularly before going to bed.

Naturopaths (who use hydrotherapy techniques) may recommend a series of hot and cold wraps to boost the immune system and fight infection.

Aromatherapy

Essential oils with antiviral properties, such as bergamot, eucalyptus, and tea tree, may help the body fight infection. Chamomile oil is useful for relieving itching, and lavender and peppermint oils have cooling properties. All of these oils can be added to the bath or diluted with a base oil and applied to the skin. Consult an aromatherapist before using essential oils on children.

Chinese herbalism

A Chinese doctor will prescribe specific herbs to rid the body of Wind-Heat and to speed the course of the disease by encouraging the development of a rash. Common prescriptions include Ju Hua (chrysanthemum flowers), Jin Yin Hua (honeysuckle flowers), and Bo He (peppermint).

MUMPS

The main symptoms of mumps are pain and swelling of the parotid (salivary) glands, located in front of the ears. One or both sides of the face may be affected. There may

THE PAROTID GLANDS
Situated above the angle of the jaw, below and in front of the ears, the parotid glands become inflamed and painful in mumps, causing facial swelling.

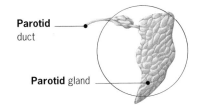
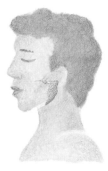

Parotid duct

Parotid gland

also be headache, fever, and difficulty in swallowing. Mumps is a viral illness that is spread by airborne droplets. Although it is usually mild, it can be uncomfortable for adult and teenage males, causing inflammation and swelling in one or both testicles and, rarely, infertility. Most children are now vaccinated against mumps in the second year of life.

There is normally a period of two to three weeks between being infected with mumps and the appearance of symptoms. There are no conventional treatments to speed up the illness, which usually runs its course in 7 to 10 days, but painkillers are sometimes prescribed to reduce discomfort. Homeopathy, Chinese herbalism, and naturopathy may relieve the symptoms of mumps and speed recovery.

Homeopathy

Rhus toxicodendron For throbbing pain that is worse on the left side of the face and is exacerbated by cold, damp weather.
Belladonna For a high temperature, a red face, and pain that is worse on the right side of the face.
Pilocarpine For severe headache and thick, sticky saliva.
Phytolacca For swollen, hard glands under the jaw and pain in the ear on swallowing.

Chinese herbalism

A decoction called Qiang Lang Tang (notopterygium and isatis root decoction) is thought to alleviate the fever, headache, pain, muscle aches, and sore throat that are associated with mumps. The remedy is believed to work by expelling Heat and toxins from the body through sweating.

Naturopathy

Restrict diet to light foods, such as clear soups, fruit juices, and fresh fruits and vegetables. Avoid dairy products, eggs, red meat, and sugar. Drink plenty of fluids.

MEASLES

A viral infection spread by airborne droplets of nasal secretion, measles symptoms are fever, runny nose, sore eyes, cough, and general malaise, followed by a rash that starts on the head and neck and spreads down the body (the rash usually subsides after three days). The glands in the neck, armpits, and groin may be swollen. Some people suffer from diarrhea and vomiting. Most children are now vaccinated against measles.

Although adults are less likely to get measles than children, it may be more serious when they do, particularly in pregnant women. Medical help should be sought if measles is suspected. Natural therapies that complement conventional treatment include homeopathy, hydrotherapy, Western and Chinese herbalism, and naturopathy.

Homeopathy

Aconite For the prerash stage of measles.
Bryonia For a rash that takes more than five days to appear, a high temperature, thirst, and a dry hacking cough accompanied by irritability.
Sulfur For a rash of purplish spots that lasts more than five days.

Hydrotherapy

The discomfort of a rash may be eased by taking warm baths with ¼ cup of baking soda or two handfuls of oatmeal added.

Herbalism

Witch hazel solution applied to the skin can relieve itching. Drinking infusions of peppermint, yarrow, or saffron may reduce fever, while taking echinacea tincture or capsules may boost the immune system.

Chinese herbalism

An herbalist will try to eliminate Wind and Heat from the body and promote the eruption of a rash. Sheng Ma Ge Gen Tang (cimifuga and kudzu decoction), which contains a mixture of red peony root and baked licorice may be prescribed.

Naturopathy

During the feverish stage of measles, a liquid diet of vegetable and fruit juices, clear soups, and water is recommended. This keeps the body hydrated and maintains strength during the most exhausting stage of the illness. After the feverish stage, eat simple foods such as fresh vegetables and fruits and whole-grain cereals.

TREATING RASHES
Witch hazel has soothing, anti-inflammatory properties. Soak a ball of cotton in witch hazel solution and apply to the affected area.

WHOOPING COUGH

Also known as pertussis, whooping cough is a bacterial infection spread by airborne droplets. The main symptom is coughing spasms that end with a "whoop" sound as breath is rapidly drawn back into the lungs. Whooping cough can last up to 10 weeks. Its complications include nosebleeds, vomiting, bleeding from the vessels on the surface of the eye, pneumonia, and collapsed lungs. If the patient has severe vomiting attacks or becomes blue through lack of oxygen, seek immediate medical help. Most children are now vaccinated against pertussis.

Antibiotics are usually prescribed, but they are not very effective unless given at the beginning of the illness. After conventional diagnosis and treatment, homeopathy, aromatherapy, Western and Chinese herbalism, and naturopathy can ease a severe cough.

Homeopathy

Drosera For a dry, tickly throat and violent cough with vomiting.
Kali carbonica For a hard, dry, hacking cough that is worse during the night.
Coccus For vomiting clear mucus and coughing eased by drinking cold water.

Aromatherapy

Try inhalations and chest rubs using black pepper, eucalyptus, tea tree, rosemary, and cypress oils. One drop of benzoin oil on the tongue daily for the first two weeks of illness may also help. Consult an aromatherapist before using essential oils on children.

Herbalism

Infusions of mullein, thyme, or horehound or a decoction of elecampane are recommended by herbalists. (Avoid thyme if you are pregnant or breast feeding.)

Chinese herbalism

An herbalist will prescribe herbs, specific to each patient, to expel Heat, phlegm, and Wind in the lungs.

Naturopathy

Honey can soothe the throat and garlic is useful for its antibacterial properties. Drink lots of water, fruit juices, and clear soups. Avoid dairy products.

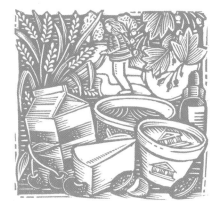

CHAPTER 7

SERIOUS AND CHRONIC CONDITIONS

*The main role of natural therapies in the
complex diseases of the heart and blood vessels,
lungs, and bones is a preventive one. Many conditions
such as hypertension and osteoporosis may be avoided
with moderate exercise, a healthy, well-balanced diet,
and giving up smoking and excessive alcohol
consumption. Even if you have a serious health
problem, adopting these measures
can lessen its severity.*

RESPIRATORY DISORDERS

Bronchitis and asthma are more serious than most common infections or allergies because the lungs become congested, causing difficult and labored breathing.

Acupressure for asthma

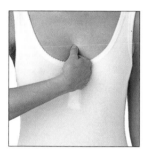

PRESSURE POINT CV 17 This is located on the center of the breastbone, three thumb widths up from the bottom of the bone.

Although conventional medical help should be sought first, natural therapies that relieve congestion in the lungs or relax tight muscles in the chest and back can help ease the symptoms of asthma and bronchitis.

BRONCHITIS

Bronchitis, an inflammation of the lining of the bronchi, is often caused by a viral or bacterial infection. It produces breathlessness and a cough with green or yellow sputum. Chronic bronchitis is associated with cigarette smoking. Conventional treatments include antibiotics, cough medicines, and inhaled drugs that dilate or widen the air passages. Sometimes pneumonia is a complication of bronchitis. If you have a fever as well as a cough and breathlessness, you should seek medical help right away.

Homeopathy, herbalism, aromatherapy, and massage may help alleviate the congestion of bronchitis.

Homeopathy
Kali carbonicum For loose, white sputum, with a rattling cough and irritability.
Pulsatilla For profuse yellow sputum.
Phosphorus For a cough and breathlessness.
Herbalism
Herbalists recommend a tincture or decoction of elecampane, or an infusion of mullein or white horehound.
Aromatherapy
Add three drops each of eucalyptus and sweet thyme oil to a bowl of hot water and inhale deeply. Avoid thyme oil during pregnancy.
Massage
A 30-minute back massage using a stroke called tapotement (see page 39) may help to loosen mucus.

ASTHMA
There may be an inherited tendency to asthma, but most attacks are provoked by food allergies (especially in children), stress, air pollution, pollen, pets, dust mites, and respiratory infections. Symptoms include breathlessness, wheezing, a tight chest, and a dry cough. The main treatment is inhaling bronchodilator drugs, which make breathing easier by widening the airways. Acupressure, reflexology, and yoga may help.
Acupressure
Apply pressure to pressure point CV 17, either to prevent the onset of an attack or to alleviate symptoms once one has begun.
Reflexology
Gently rub the skin between the big toe and the second toe—asthmatics often find this area quite tender.
Yoga
Stress and anxiety can increase your breathing rate, exacerbating symptoms of asthma. Yoga can help (see opposite).

THE SYMPTOMS OF BRONCHITIS Whether you suffer from acute or chronic bronchitis, your principal symptoms will be wheezing, coughing, and breathlessness.

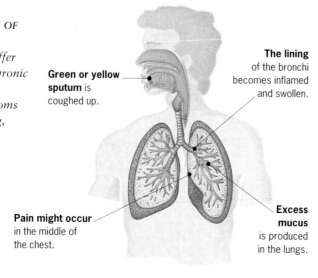

Green or yellow sputum is coughed up.

The lining of the bronchi becomes inflamed and swollen.

Pain might occur in the middle of the chest.

Excess mucus is produced in the lungs.

Breathing Difficulties

Although it is not a cure for bronchitis or asthma, yoga can help ease symptoms through deep breathing techniques, which ease tense muscles, reduce stress levels, and promote relaxation.

To reap the full benefits of yoga, you should be taught by an experienced teacher. Many poses, however, are easy to practice at home. Find a quiet place in a warm, well-ventilated room. Wear comfortable, loose clothing or workout clothing that does not restrict your movements. Yoga is best practiced before a meal or at least two hours after eating.

Although yoga may appear to be straightforward, its apparent simplicity is deceptive—the exercises require careful control of muscles, posture, and breathing.

DEEP RELAXATION
Lie on your back and inhale and exhale, concentrating on the sensation your breathing creates. Imagine your abdomen expanding and collapsing like a balloon.

EXERCISES TO EASE BREATHLESSNESS

One of the main symptoms of asthma and bronchitis is breathlessness. Yoga can help by teaching you deep breathing techniques.

DEEP RELAXATION
You can practice deep breathing while relaxing by lying on your back and concentrating on the physical sensation of your body on the floor. Feel the rising and falling movements of your abdomen, filling and emptying like a balloon as you breathe. Let the breath flow in and out naturally, without trying to control it. Count 10 breaths, noting how the movements become increasingly regular. Next, feel yourself energized by the incoming air when you inhale and feel yourself relax as you exhale. Imagine your body sinking into the floor as your abdomen falls, and then becoming light and energetic as your abdomen rises.

ARM-STRETCH BREATHING
Stand with your feet apart, holding your arms out in front of you with your palms touching. Slowly inhale, spreading your arms sideways and slightly back so that your chest expands. As you exhale, bring your arms back to the front.

THE COBRA
Lie on your stomach with your head on the floor and your legs together. Your elbows should be bent so that your hands are flat on the floor and your fingertips align with your shoulders. Now, slowly inhale and raise your head from the floor. Exhale. Inhale again, this time raising your chest off the floor, without pushing on your arms. Now exhale. Inhale, but this time press down on the floor and lift your chest as far up as you can, stopping just before your navel comes off the floor.

ARM-STRETCH BREATHING
Stand straight with your legs relaxed and your feet slightly apart. Inhale as you spread your arms apart. Repeat five times.

THE COBRA
Hold this position for three to five breaths, then return to lying flat on the floor, breathing out as you do so.

CARDIOVASCULAR DISEASES

Some diseases of the heart and blood vessels can be controlled by changes in lifestyle. The focus of natural therapies is on a healthy diet and exercise, plus stress reduction and relaxation.

*PSYCHOFEEDBACK
This computer software is one advance in biofeedback technology. Electrodes measuring electrodermal activity (an indication of emotional state) are attached to your fingers. The screen image changes as you become more relaxed.*

Hypertension (persistently high blood pressure) and heart disease are life threatening, so it is essential that you receive the correct diagnosis and treatment from your doctor before you try natural remedies. The role of natural therapies is to prevent problems or to complement—not replace—conventional treatments.

HYPERTENSION

Blood pressure refers to the force blood exerts on the arteries of the heart as it is pumped throughout the body. Regulated by hormones and nerve sensors, blood pressure varies according to age and activity. When blood pressure levels remain consistently elevated, hypertension is diagnosed.

Hypertension is sometimes called the silent killer because it is usually symptomless and remains undiagnosed until detected during a routine examination. If left untreated, it may lead to kidney damage, heart failure, or stroke. Conventional treatment includes drugs that lower the heart rate, dilate blood vessels, or eliminate fluids.

There are several lifestyle changes that are effective in lowering blood pressure. If you smoke, give it up immediately. Make sure that your weight is within standard guidelines—obese people are at greater risk of hypertension. Even if you are not overweight, try to reduce the amount of fat, alcohol, and salt in your diet. You should also make time for regular, moderate exercise.

Among the natural remedies that can help reduce hypertension are Chinese herbalism and biofeedback. The naturopathic remedies for heart disease (see opposite page) may also help to reduce hypertension.

Chinese herbalism

Celery seed is a Western herb that Chinese doctors use to treat hypertension. Consult a Chinese herbalist for an individual prescription. Avoid celery seed if you are pregnant.

Biofeedback

Stress can be an aggravating factor in hypertension. Studies reported in the *British Medical Journal* in 1988 showed that practicing the techniques learned in biofeedback led to reduced stress levels and lower blood pressure in people who had hypertension.

By monitoring normally unconscious body activities like muscle tension, skin temperature, or pulse rate, biofeedback machines can teach you to modify your physical response to stress. One type of biofeedback involves a temperature sensor attached to a finger. Because your hands become colder as anxiety levels increase, they indicate how tense you're feeling. Another type, Psychofeedback, is computer software that uses visual images to show how stressed or relaxed you are. You can learn to respond to a machine's indicators by relaxing with such techniques as creative visualization, deep breathing, and meditation. As you become familiar with your body's responses to stress, you can eventually use these techniques to lower blood pressure without the aid of a biofeedback machine.

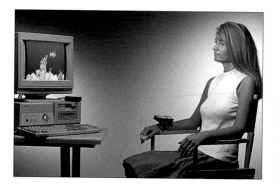

HEART DISEASE AND STROKE

The leading cause of death in the United States is cardiovascular disease, which includes atherosclerosis, angina, heart attack, and stroke. A diet high in saturated fat and lack of exercise (among other things) may lead to atherosclerosis by causing a clogging of the arteries with cholesterol-rich fatty deposits. As a result, blood supply is restricted, and parts of the heart may become temporarily short of blood, causing angina (severe pain in the chest following exercise or stress).

If deterioration of the blood flow continues and a coronary artery becomes blocked, a heart attack occurs. A stroke occurs when blood flow to the brain is interrupted or there is a leakage of blood into the brain due to a ruptured artery. A severe heart attack or stroke may be fatal.

Conventional treatment for heart disease and stroke is drug based. Sometimes surgery is recommended to repair or replace damaged arteries. The following therapies may help prevent cardiovascular disease.

Herbalism

The following tonic is thought to be useful for any heart disorder. Mix equal amounts of linden flowers and hawthorn berries, and make an infusion (use 1 teaspoon of each of the dried herbs to every cup of water). Take half a teaspoonful of the liquid three times a day. Fresh garlic and some brands of garlic capsules can help lower blood cholesterol levels.

Chinese medicine

Therapy usually involves a combination of herbalism and acupuncture. Treatment can be preventive or it can alleviate the symptoms of an existing heart condition. Herbal remedies are tailored to fit your individual requirements; you'll probably need to take them for several months.

In China, acupuncture is often used to treat minor strokes, and acupuncturists claim good recovery rates. The findings of clinical trials performed in Scandinavia support these claims. Treatment should start as soon after a stroke as possible and should continue throughout rehabilitation.

Naturopathy

A low-fat vegetarian diet may help reduce blood cholesterol and prevent cardiovascular problems. Fish oils, which contain omega-3 fatty acids, are believed to help to reduce your risk of heart disease by lowering your blood pressure and your blood cholesterol levels. Try to eat oily fish such as mackerel or tuna one to three times a week. If this is not possible, fish oils are also available in capsules. Vitamins B (especially B_6), C, and E and magnesium are thought to have a positive impact on heart disease.

HOW MUCH EXERCISE DO YOU GET?

Exercise is vital to maintaining cardiovascular health. Any exercise is better than none, but working out vigorously three times a week for at least 20 minutes is recommended. Your pulse should reach 60 to 75 percent of your maximum heart rate, which is determined by subtracting your age from 220. As much as possible, include exercise in your daily life.

▶ *Walk rather than drive to work and other destinations.*

▶ *Use stairs instead of an elevator*

▶ *Regularly schedule active leisure-time activities, such as tennis, bowling, biking, or golf.*

DIET AND THE HEALTH OF YOUR HEART

High consumption of saturated fat is one reason that some people develop heart disease. You can dramatically reduce your risk of cardiovascular illness by changing your dietary habits. Eat less red meat, high-fat dairy products, and processed foods, and more fish, fruits, and vegetables. Drink skim milk instead of whole.

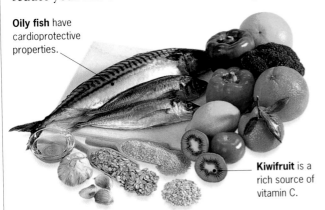

Oily fish have cardioprotective properties.

Kiwifruit is a rich source of vitamin C.

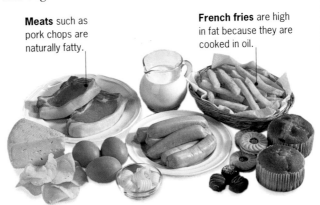

Meats such as pork chops are naturally fatty.

French fries are high in fat because they are cooked in oil.

FOODS YOU SHOULD EAT
Fish oils, garlic, vitamin C, and foods rich in water-soluble fiber, such as citrus fruits, potatoes, and cereal brans, can lower cholesterol levels and reduce the risk of heart disease.

FOODS TO AVOID
The fat on pork chops is obvious; other foods, such as cookies, may contain invisible fat. Steamed, roasted, or broiled foods are better than fried foods.

The Workaholic

Devoting too much time and energy to your job may be a subconscious attempt to ignore personal issues that you find hard to deal with. Also, if you spend most of your days and evenings at work, you may be neglecting your health because you will have little time for a well-balanced diet, adequate exercise, and relaxation.

Paul is 41 years old and has worked at a large advertising agency for 10 years. Two years ago his wife, Helen, died of breast cancer. Paul has two children: a 22-year-old son, Mark, who lives away from home, and an 18-year-old daughter, Vicky, who is a senior in high school.

Paul works extremely hard and his colleagues admire him, but many think he's a workaholic, especially since Helen's death. This has left him with virtually no time for himself or to spend with his children or friends.

When Paul's wife died, he appeared to cope admirably—his approach was to put on a brave face and carry on as normal. Vicky, however, felt that her father was too unemotional and she resents the fact that she has never been able to talk openly to him about her mother's death. She is also unhappy that her father spends so little time at home, and this has led to tension between them.

Paul believes he's in good health, but he often suffers from fatigue and feels irritable and unable to concentrate. At the end of the day, he unwinds by drinking whiskey and smoking. At a company medical examination, Paul is told that his blood pressure is high, that he is overweight, and that his workaholic tendencies may lead to chronic fatigue. (Paul's previous medical check-ups have revealed mild hypertension.) Paul is told that he needs to start taking blood pressure medication, particularly since he has a family history of cardiovascular disease.

Paul realizes that he needs to look at how he can prevent his health from deteriorating, and how he can improve his relationship with Vicky.

FAMILY
A breakdown in communications among family members, especially in the aftermath of a major life event such as the death of a loved one, can cause some resentment and hostility.

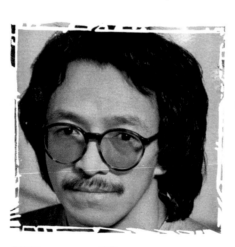

HEALTH
A poor diet, cigarette smoking, too much alcohol, and too little exercise are all risk factors for diseases affecting circulation, the heart, and the blood vessels.

BEREAVEMENT
People who are grieving may appear to be coping, but suppressed feelings can surface later in physical or pyschological illness.

WORK
Working long hours can become a habit and may lead to chronic stress—a risk factor for cardiovascular disease.

LIFESTYLE
Spending little or no time relaxing and neglecting personal relationships can lead to emotional and physical ill health.

WHAT PAUL SHOULD DO

The amount of time he spends at work and the nature of his work are causing Paul's chronic stress. He needs to find ways of decreasing his workload and relaxing more. He should also consider why he took on such a heavy workload in the first place and how it may be linked to the death of his wife. By adopting what he thought was a "strong" role and immersing himself in work, Paul may have prevented his own recovery. Although Helen died two years ago, both Paul and Vicky would benefit from seeing a bereavement counselor. This would also help them reestablish their once strong relationship.

Paul needs to take his high blood pressure very seriously and find ways to reduce it. Cutting back on his workload will decrease his overall stress level, but Paul also needs to give up smoking and find alternatives to alcohol to help him relax. Taking up an exercise such as swimming not only will help bring Paul's weight down but also improve his cardiovascular fitness and self-esteem. Massage, yoga, or meditation, will also be beneficial.

Hypertension can be reduced by maintaining a healthy diet—Paul should try to minimize the amount of saturated fat and salt in his diet and start to eat more fruits, vegetables, beans, and whole grains.

Action Plan

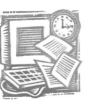

FAMILY
Reduce working hours to spend more time at home with Vicky. Arrange to visit Mark and perhaps suggest a family outing or vacation.

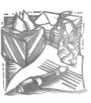

LIFESTYLE
Leave space in daily routine for relaxation, meal planning, and free time. Go swimming a couple of times a week. Think about contacting old friends and rebuilding a social life.

WORK
Look at workload, prioritize jobs, and discuss delegating work with boss. Stop working late and on weekends and make a concerted effort to forget about work when out of the office.

BEREAVEMENT
Talk to Vicky about attending some sessions together with a bereavement counselor. Try to spend time talking to Vicky about her feelings.

HEALTH
Arrange sessions with a massage therapist and listen to relaxation tapes at home. Substitute healthy food for high-fat, low-fiber processed food, and reduce salt intake. Try to give up smoking and cut down on alcohol.

HOW THINGS TURNED OUT FOR PAUL

Simply by working normal hours, Paul managed to organize his life better. He began to spend more time with Vicky and his diet improved: he now eats fewer foods that are high in saturated fat and more that are high in fiber.

At first Paul felt that his job might be in jeopardy because he was not putting in enough hours, but this feeling soon abated, although he occasionally feels threatened by younger colleagues.

Paul tried practicing relaxation techniques at home but he couldn't keep it up. However, his weekly massage sessions have helped him relax. He swims on weekends and finds time to go for walks, a pastime he discovered he enjoys and can share with Vicky. He also managed to cut down on smoking and drinking.

Vicky and Paul attended three sessions with a bereavement counselor, where they inititiated

discussions about Helen's death and its impact on them. There is less tension between them, and Vicky understands that her father's silence was his way of dealing with his feelings.

Paul's blood pressure is reduced, but he still needs to take medication to bring it down to safe levels. He feels very confident about his progress and hopes to have his blood pressure back to normal within a year.

MUSCULOSKELETAL DISORDERS

Diseases of the bones, muscles, and joints can be very painful and debilitating. In severe cases, even simple movements such as getting out of a chair can become difficult.

Sufferers of joint and muscle pain can benefit greatly from a number of natural therapies, both ancient and modern.

ARTHRITIS

Arthritis is the medical term for any disease that produces inflammation, pain, and stiffness in one or more joints. There are many different types, all classified as rheumatic diseases. An approach that combines medication, exercise, and rest is basic to the conventional treatment of most forms. Natural therapies aim to relieve discomfort.

Homeopathy
Colchicum For inflamed joints that worsen in warm weather.
Rhus toxicodendron For stiff joints that are worse after rest, or in the cold or damp.

Herbalism
A surprising ancient treatment for arthritis that many people find effective today is the application of stinging nettle leaves to the inflamed joints; the leaves must be handled with gloves, but are quite effective in bringing relief. Nettle leaves can also be boiled and eaten as a vegetable, or the cooking water taken as a tea. Other herbs useful for arthritis include dandelion, taken as a tea, chamomile, boiled and applied with a compress, and evening primrose, in capsule form.

If the arthritic joint feels cold, try applying a liniment of equal parts of tincture of cayenne and glycerin. Do not use it on broken skin and test it first on a small patch of skin.

Aromatherapy
Add a few drops of lavender, marjoram, peppermint, or rosemary essential oil to a base oil. Rub into the skin around the joint.

Hydrotherapy
The pain of osteoarthritis can often be relieved with warm, moist compresses applied for 10 to 15 minutes every few hours. Another approach, which may relieve pain by increasing circulation to the affected area, is to alternately apply hot compresses (for 2 minutes) and cold compresses (for 30 seconds). Also, try your exercise regimen in a heated swimming pool. Underwater movement is gentler to the joints than working out on a hard surface.

Naturopathy
Oily fish contains omega-3 fatty acids, which are thought to inhibit inflammation; vitamin E, found in nuts and wheat germ, may also help. Some arthritis sufferers have found relief by eliminating all animal foods, including dairy products, from their diets. There is also some indication that food sensitivities may trigger arthritic symptoms.

HAND MASSAGE FOR ARTHRITIS

When giving a massage, avoid applying pressure to a painful arthritic joint—instead, apply strokes to the area immediately above and below the swelling. Lubricate the skin using marjoram essential oil diluted with a base oil.

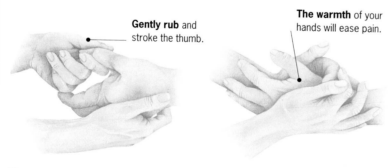

Gently rub and stroke the thumb.

The warmth of your hands will ease pain.

THUMB MASSAGE
Using your thumb and finger, apply gentle stroking movements to the area around the site of the pain.

WHOLE HAND MASSAGE
Enclose the sufferer's hand in both of your hands and stroke from the wrist to the fingertips.

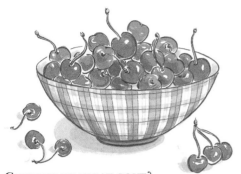

CHERRIES TO TREAT GOUT?
Some people say that eating cherries every day will lower uric-acid levels and prevent gout attacks, but there is little evidence for this claim.

GOUT

Gout is a painful condition caused by a build-up of uric acid crystals that become lodged in certain areas of the body, usually the first joint of the big toe. This common disease mainly affects adult males. The main symptoms are inflammation and intense pain.

Sufferers may experience one acute episode of gout or repeated attacks. If left untreated, the joints may become damaged. Also, chronic gout causes the buildup of uric acid crystals in the kidneys, causing kidney stones, kidney failure, or high blood pressure. Conventional treatments for gout are anti-inflammatory drugs or medications that increase the excretion of uric acid. The natural remedies for gout include herbalism, reflexology, homeopathy, and naturopathy.

Herbalism
An infusion of equal parts of burdock root, celery seed, and yarrow may help relieve pain. Drink the infusion three times a day. Avoid celery seed during pregnancy.

Reflexology
If one or both of your big toes are affected by gout, try massaging the thumb joint where it joins the hand on the side opposite the painful toe. Repeat this frequently.

Homeopathy
Belladonna For a joint that is painful, red, and tender and made worse by touching.
Arnica For a joint that aches or feels as though it has been bruised.

Naturopathy
Charcoal tablets, taken four times a day, may reduce uric acid levels. Drinking three quarts of water a day helps to flush out your system. Foods that contain crystalline compounds called purines should be avoided because purines are converted to uric acid in the body. Red meat, shellfish, oily fish (especially anchovies and sardines), and alcoholic and caffeinated beverages contain purines.

CHRONIC FATIGUE SYNDROME
The varying symptoms of this debilitating condition include extreme exhaustion, muscle aches and pains, headaches, digestive problems, breathing difficulties, poor concentration, depression, and speech problems.

Although it is sometimes precipitated by a viral infection, such as influenza, the exact cause of chronic fatigue syndrome (CFS) is unknown. Instead of recovering from a viral infection in a few days, the CFS sufferer will continue to feel weak and debilitated for weeks or months. It is thought that emotional or physical stress may also cause CFS.

CFS has only recently been recognized by the medical establishment and it is often diagnosed by a process of elimination. Conventional treatment consists of rest, painkillers, anti-inflammatory drugs, and antidepressants. Homeopathy, Bach flower remedies, and naturopathy may help.

Homeopathy
Cases of CFS have responded well to homeopathic remedies. Because the symptoms of CFS are so diverse, you should consult a homeopath for an individual prescription.

Bach flower remedies
Olive is recommended for fatigue and feeling drained of energy, and wild rose may alleviate feelings of depression and apathy.

Naturopathy
A CFS sufferer may have a food intolerance, such as one for lactose, or an allergy (see page 66), and this should be investigated by a naturopath or dietitian. Nicotine and foods that contain sugar, alcohol, and caffeine are thought to exacerbate symptoms of CFS; they should be avoided.

Because food absorption in some CFS sufferers may be impaired, several small meals during the day may be better than one or two large meals.

continued on page 108

READY-TO-EAT SNACKS
If you suffer from CFS and find it hard to eat large meals, eat small amounts frequently. Healthy snacks such as fruit, cheese, whole-wheat crackers, nuts, and raisins are beneficial.

The Dietitian

If you are at risk for osteoporosis, it is important to consult a dietitian. This specialist can give you not only advice about specific foods you should eat but also, if necessary, supplements to take.

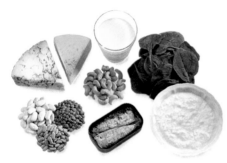

CALCIUM-RICH FOODS
Dairy products, beans, leafy green vegetables, and fish with soft, digestible bones, such as sardines, are excellent sources of calcium.

CONSULTING A DIETITIAN
A dietitian will take a detailed history of your dietary habits. This information will help her to suggest some appropriate changes.

A dietitian specializes in nutrition and has knowledge of chemistry, biology, physiology, and micro-biology. The American Dietetic Association awards the Registered Dietitian credential to those who pass a certification examination after completing a bachelor's degree program and supervised work experience. In addition, many states have license or certification requirements.

When should I visit a dietitian?
It is generally accepted that a healthy diet can go a long way to relieve and prevent many conditions. If you or your doctor is able to pinpoint specific areas of your diet that may

be responsible for ill health, or if you feel that your diet is lacking in certain areas, a dietitian will be able to give you advice.

Will my doctor refer me to a dietitian?
General advice on diet will not need a doctor's referral. For specific disorders, for example gastrointestinal disorders, the dietitian may require information from your doctor. In some cases your doctor may recommend that you seek specific dietary guidance. For an overview, such as general guidelines for a high-calcium diet, you can approach a dietitian directly. You can find one through your doctor or local health center.

How can a dietitian help with osteoporosis?
Dietitians recommend getting an adequate amount of calcium throughout your lifetime. A calcium-rich diet is particularly important during childhood, adolescence, and early adulthood, in order to establish an optimum peak bone mass (PBM). Insufficient calcium intake may mean that your bones do not reach their optimum mass, and you will be more likely to suffer from brittle bones in the future. After you have reached your PBM in your late twenties, it's still important that you continue to consume adequate calcium.

How can a low-fat diet include calcium-rich dairy products?
Low-fat dairy products are the answer. One cup (8 fluid ounces) of skim milk contains more calcium

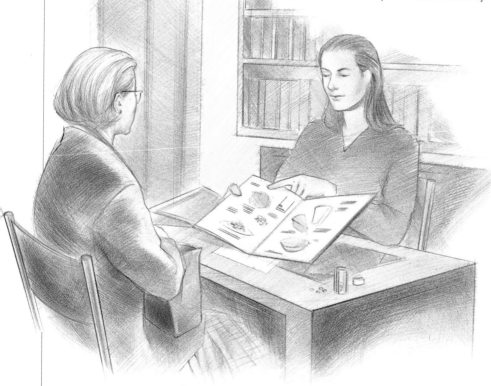

than the same amount of whole milk (296 milligrams and 288 milligrams respectively). A 1½-ounce slice of reduced-fat hard cheese contains more calcium than ordinary Cheddar (335 milligrams compared with 300 milligrams). Low-fat yogurt is an excellent source of calcium.

Do any foods deplete calcium?
Some types of fiber, found mostly in cereal bran and whole grains, may deplete calcium. Therefore, you should avoid eating excessive amounts of bran and unleavened breads such as matzo (other breads, even whole-wheat, do not deplete calcium because of their yeast content). High intakes of protein, phosphorus, or caffeine may also deplete calcium from the body. Smoking cigarettes and excess alcohol consumption may inhibit calcium absorption.

Why do I need more calcium after menopause?
Bone loss is accelerated for the first five years after menopause because the ovaries greatly reduce the production of estrogen (estrogen is essential for the absorption of calcium into the bones), so it is important to keep up your calcium intake. The National Osteoporosis Foundation recommends 1,500 milligrams of calcium a day for postmenopausal women. The recommended calcium intake for premenopausal women is 1,000 milligrams per day.

Does hormone replacement therapy affect calcium requirements?
Taking supplementary estrogen in the form of hormone replacement therapy (HRT) will protect your bones from excessive mineral loss so extra calcium is not necessary. The National Osteoporosis Foundation recommends 1,000 milligrams of calcium a day if you are taking HRT. Speak to your doctor about the degree of protection offered by the form of HRT that you are taking.

Which calcium supplement is best?
Dietitians recommend chewable or effervescent calcium supplements, such as calcium lactate or gluconate, which are better absorbed than other supplements because they dissolve more easily in the stomach. This makes the calcium more readily available for absorption and is better suited to older people who may absorb calcium less efficiently. At 40 percent, calcium carbonate contains the highest concentration of calcium.

Are calcium supplements safe for everyone?
Consult your doctor before taking supplements if you are prone to kidney stones, have kidney disease, or are anemic, because too much calcium can interfere with iron

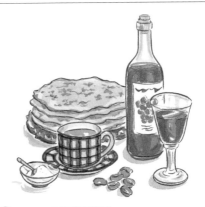

CALCIUM DEPLETERS
An excess of caffeine, alcohol, high-protein foods, bran, and sodium can reduce your body's calcium levels.

absorption. If you are taking diuretics or antibiotics, it is a good idea to ask your doctor's advice about the possible side effects of taking calcium supplements at the same time.

WHAT YOU CAN DO AT HOME

Keep a diary of the meals you eat over a period of a week and check to see how many of them are rich in calcium. If you find that you eat very few dairy products, leafy green vegetables, canned fish with soft bones, and beans, it is likely that your calcium intake is low. Plan breakfast, lunch, and dinner menus that incorporate these foods, making sure that you eat at least one calcium-rich meal a day, and drink skim milk.

BREAKFAST
Oatmeal made with skim milk and a little butter on your toast can boost your calcium intake at breakfast.

LUNCH
A glass of skim milk plus low-fat yogurt on a baked potato can add calcium to a midday meal.

DINNER
Vegetarian lasagna with a low-fat cheese topping and fruit pie with a little custard make a high-calcium evening meal.

HIGH-RISK FACTORS FOR OSTEOPOROSIS

Various factors can cause a low peak bone mass leading to osteoporosis. If one or more of the following applies to you, and you are in your fifties or sixties, ask your doctor about having a bone density scan.

▶ *A diet that lacks sufficient calcium.*
▶ *Amenorrhea (absence of menstruation).*
▶ *Long-term treatment with diuretics or thyroid hormones.*
▶ *Surgical removal of the ovaries or a premature menopause.*
▶ *Cigarette smoking.*
▶ *Little or no weight-bearing exercise in your twenties and thirties.*
▶ *Treatment with corticosteroids (for rheumatoid arthritis).*
▶ *A family history of osteoporosis.*

COPING WITH CFS

Because CFS can be a long-term disease, it is important to have strategies to cope with exhaustion. Include rest periods in your daily routine and make sure that your family, friends, and colleagues understand the reason for your tiredness. Try not to travel long distances, and allow yourself double the normal time to do everyday tasks. Don't be self-critical when you are restricted by fatigue. Reduce work and domestic commitments to the bare minimum and learn to relax and conserve energy. Combat stress with therapies such as meditation, yoga, or tai chi.

Scientific studies suggest that evening primrose oil and magnesium, taken over time, can alleviate the symptoms of CFS. In clinical trials, 1/10 ounce of evening primrose oil was taken every day and intramuscular injections of magnesium were given. Consult a naturopath about this.

Many naturopaths believe that chronic candida (yeast) infections are responsible for the digestive symptoms such as bloating and diarrhea that are typical of CFS. To combat this, they recommend a sugar-free diet and high doses of vitamin C. If you are suffering from CFS and experience severe digestive symptoms, seek advice from a doctor or naturopath about elimination diets (do not attempt them on your own).

OSTEOPOROSIS

Osteoporosis is an age-related disease that is caused by a loss of bone mass, most often resulting from insufficient calcium. It causes the bones to become thin, porous, and prone to fracture. Common fracture sites are the hip, thigh, wrist, and spine. Compression fractures in the spine, which cause back pain, decreased height, and "dowager's hump"—a rounding of the upper part of the back, occur when the vertebrae collapse onto each other.

Osteoporosis is most common in postmenopausal women. The female hormone estrogen is vital for the body's absorption of calcium, but after menopause the production of estrogen diminishes. Therefore, one way to prevent osteoporosis is to maintain estrogen levels with hormone replacement therapy (HRT). Such treatment is also effective in checking existing osteoporosis and limiting further damage. Injections or a nasal spray of calcitonin, a calcium-regulating hormone, are also available for women who are at high risk for osteoporosis, but choose not to take HRT.

A lifelong diet high in calcium and regular weight-bearing exercise are important aspects of osteoporosis prevention. Although the first line of treatment should be orthodox medicine, therapies such as Chinese medicine may bring relief from the pain of fractures that occur with osteoporosis.

Naturopathy

Once bone mass has been lost, a calcium-rich diet will not restore it, but it will help prevent further loss. From childhood on, eating foods containing the right vitamins and minerals is an important step in preventing osteoporosis.

Calcium is essential for strong bones, but it cannot be absorbed by the body unless it is accompanied by vitamin D. Vitamin D is found in fish oil and it is generated by exposure to sunlight. An excellent source of both calcium and vitamin D is found in sardines—vitamin D is present in the flesh and calcium is present in the bones.

Smoking cigarettes and drinking alcoholic and caffeinated beverages are all associated with increased bone loss.

Chinese medicine

Acupuncture may relieve pain by increasing the output of enkephalins and endorphins, the body's natural painkillers. Chinese herbs such as Dang Gui (*Angelica sinensis*) and Du Zhong (eucomia bark) may also be prescribed by a Chinese herbalist. Herbs may be taken as infusions or tablets.

Exercise

Along with adequate calcium intake, the best way to prevent osteoporosis is through regular exercise. This is particularly important when you are in your twenties and thirties, before your bones reach their peak mass. However, at all ages, a program of 40 to 60 minutes of weight-bearing exercise, four times a week, will enable your body to retain calcium in the skeletal system. Brisk walking, jogging, skipping rope, gymnastics, tennis, aerobics, racquetball, rowing, and weight training are good forms of exercise. Consult your doctor before exercising if you are out of shape or have heart problems.

CHAPTER 8

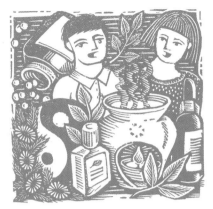

EMOTIONAL HEALTH

*In addition to painful feelings associated
with trauma and grief, stress can affect both
physical and emotional well-being. Conventional
treatment for acute stress as well as psychological
problems often includes tranquilizers or antidepressants, neither of which can be used long-term.
Among natural remedies that can help you
regain control are deep breathing and other
relaxation techniques and counseling.*

EVERYDAY LIFE

Daily problems can cause nervous tension and irritability, which may become chronic if you don't take time to relax and unwind. Natural remedies such as yoga and meditation can help.

The sources of stress and anxiety in everyday life are numerous. Problems with work, family, finances, and personal relationships can all deplete your emotional reserves, making you prone to insomnia and fatigue.

IRRITABILITY

Being short-tempered or easily angered is a natural emotional and physiological response to events that seem threatening. Irritability can be due to depression, fatigue, or the pressure of multiple responsibilities; it can also be a symptom of premenstrual tension. Feeling irritable can increase your pulse rate, put a knot in your stomach, and make your muscles tense up.

It is unlikely that a doctor will prescribe a drug for irritability, but he may question you about underlying stresses and strains, advise you to get enough rest, and perhaps ask you to try some relaxation techniques. Such therapies as yoga, herbalism, homeopathy, massage, and exercise may make you easier to live with.

RELAXING WITH YOGA

If you are feeling irritable, anxious, or tired, the following yoga pose may help. Start by sitting with your legs alongside a wall, then slide your legs up the wall so that your back is flat on the floor and your legs are at right angles to your body. Let your hands rest, relaxed, on your abdomen. Relax and breathe evenly for 5 to 10 minutes and then come out of the position in reverse order.

THE BRACKET POSE
Lying on your back with your legs against a wall relaxes tense muscles and invigorates by stimulating blood flow.

Herbalism
A limeflower infusion can help reduce tension. Herbalists may prescribe vervain or, if fatigue is the underlying problem, an all-purpose tonic.

Homeopathy
Lycopodium For irritability, touchiness, sudden outbursts of anger, and a lack of self-confidence.
Silica For people who are irritable, nervous, stubborn, and exhausted.
Nux vomica For those who are irritable, impatient, and critical.

Massage
Sit the person to be massaged in a straight-backed chair. Place your hands, palms down, on the top of the shoulders near the neck. Your touch should be firm and reassuring. Leave one hand resting on one shoulder, while you concentrate on the other. Start by using your thumb and fingers to make gentle circular movements on the muscles. Then lightly knead and squeeze them. Gradually work along the shoulder to the shoulder joint. Repeat the process on the other shoulder. End the massage by gently stroking the arm from the top of the shoulders to the fingertips three or four times.

Exercise
Regular exercise will increase your energy levels and relieve built-up anger. Try to go for a 20-minute swim, jog, or walk at least three times a week.

NERVOUS TENSION

Emotional exhaustion and nervous tension are usually caused by an inability to cope with life's pressures. They are characterized by an inability to concentrate or complete a task, and may be accompanied by fatigue, insomnia, or anxiety.

Depending on the severity of the problem, a doctor may simply recommend rest and some time off from work, with or without counseling. In very severe cases of nervous tension, drugs such as benzodiazepines and beta-blockers (antianxiety drugs) may also be prescribed to promote mental and physical relaxation, but only for definite anxiety states and only for a short time because these drugs can be addictive.

The natural treatments for nervous tension include herbalism, Bach flower remedies and aromatherapy to calm and restore the nervous system.

Herbalism
Infusions of wood betony, lavender, chamomile, and lemon balm may all help calm the nervous system.

Bach flower remedies
The Bach flower remedies for nervous tension are cherry plum for uncontrolled, irrational thoughts; gorse for hopelessness; and hornbeam for procrastination.

Aromatherapy
Essential oils that may be useful for nervous tension are bergamot, chamomile, juniper, neroli, rose, and sandalwood. Use them in a massage by mixing with a base oil or add five to eight drops to a warm bath. You can also add five to eight drops to a bowl of steaming water, put a towel over your head and the bowl, and inhale the vapors.

INSOMNIA
Problems with getting to sleep or staying asleep are common—one in three adults suffers from insomnia at some time. Insomnia is often associated with irritability and fatigue during the day.

The most common cause of insomnia is anxiety. Other causes include snoring, noise, caffeine, inactivity during the day, or keeping erratic hours. Sleeplessness can also be associated with depression, misuse of sleeping pills, or withdrawal from drugs such as antidepressants or narcotics.

Self-help measures—exercising during the day, going to bed at the same time every night, reducing alcohol and caffeine intake, and taking a warm bath before going to bed —should be tried before taking sleeping pills. Make sure that your bedroom is conducive to sleep; it should be dark, well ventilated, quiet, and warm.

Aromatherapy, Western and Chinese herbalism, and acupuncture are useful for general relaxation. Tai chi and yoga can help you to relax and get a good night's sleep by relieving stress and anxiety.

AN HERBAL SLEEPING POTION
Make an infusion with 2 teaspoons dried passionflower, 1 teaspoon dried valerian or chamomile flowers, and 1 cup water; drink it one-half to one hour before going to bed. (Avoid passionflower during pregnancy, as it may stimulate the uterine muscles.)

TAKING THE INFUSION
You can make this infusion in bulk. Store it in the refrigerator and drink one cup before you go to bed at night.

Aromatherapy
Lavender oil added to your bath or placed on your pillow and inhaled during the night may help you relax. A rosemary oil bath may raise your spirits if you feel depressed.

Herbalism
A warm bath that contains a few drops of lavender oil can warm and relax you. A tea made with lavender, catnip, the combination above, or hops can also be effective. (Avoid hops if you suffer from depression.) Try also the mustard footbath described at right.

Yoga
If you cannot get to sleep, try the following yoga pose for five minutes. Take a chair and place it in front of you. Sit on a cushion or folded blanket with your legs straight out in front of you under the chair, then lean forward as if to touch your toes and rest your head and arms on the seat of the chair. Keeping your legs straight, relax your body, neck, arms, and head and breathe deeply and slowly. Concentrate on your breathing and clear your mind of all other thoughts.

Tai chi
The flowing movements of tai chi help the body's energy to flow freely, allowing you to relax. You should go to a qualified teacher to learn the correct series of movements. You will soon be familiar with the movements and able to practice every day.

Chinese medicine
If Liver Fire is thought to cause your insomnia, a Chinese herbalist may prescribe Long Dan Xie Gan Tang (Chinese gentian root drain the Liver decoction). For Heart and Spleen Blood deficiency, Gui Pi Tang (restore the Spleen decoction) may be prescribed. Acupuncturists use points to tone the Heart and Spleen or calm the Liver and mind.

Mustard footbath for insomnia
If you have trouble getting to sleep, try soaking your feet in a warming mustard footbath before you go to bed each night.

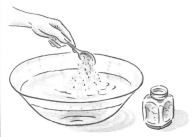

PREPARING A FOOTBATH
Add 1 heaping tablespoon of mustard powder to a large bowl of hot water.

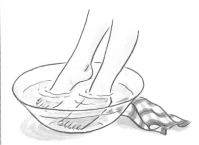

SOAKING YOUR FEET
Immerse your feet in the mustard and water mixture for 15 minutes every night.

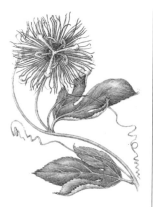

PASSIONFLOWER
The sedative properties of passionflower make it useful for calming the nervous system and promoting sleep. (Avoid passion-flower during pregnancy.)

FATIGUE

Everyone goes through periods in their life when they feel tired, listless, and disinterested in people and the world around them. Fatigue has many causes, both physical and emotional. Physical causes include low blood sugar, an underactive thyroid gland, anemia, chronic fatigue syndrome (see page 105), mononucleosis (see page 94), and pregnancy. Emotional causes include stress, anxiety, repressed emotions, and depression. When fatigue is the only complaint, the cause is likely to be psychological (stress, anxiety, emotional trauma). The longer it lasts without other symptoms, the more likely it is to be depression.

Conventional medical treatment for fatigue consists of treating any underlying physiological cause. For example, if an underactive thyroid gland were diagnosed, it would be treated with the drug thyroxin. If fatigue is associated with depression, your doctor may prescribe antidepressants.

Natural remedies for fatigue include acupressure, relaxation techniques, and Chinese herbalism.

Acupressure

If you are feeling run-down, try pressing St 36 (see page 128), four finger widths down from the base of the kneecap on the outside of the leg. Applying pressure to Sp 6 (see page 128), three finger widths up from the inner ankle bone, may also help alleviate fatigue (avoid applying pressure to this point during pregnancy).

Relaxation

Rest is vital to recover from fatigue. Make sure you get enough sleep and go to bed at a regular time every night. Get help around the house and at work and try not to take on any extra responsibilities. If possible, try to take a vacation for a week or two to recover fully. Spend time doing whatever you find relaxing: swimming, reading, going for a walk, or listening to music. Practicing yoga may help.

The child's pose is a yoga position that helps alleviate fatigue caused by stress and anxiety by helping you to relax tense muscles and clear your mind. To adopt the child's pose, lie on a mat or towel with your knees drawn up beneath you and out to the sides. With your arms by your side, your head should rest on the floor. Relax your muscles and breathe slowly, completely filling and emptying your lungs with each breath.

Chinese herbalism

Chinese medicine regards exhaustion as due to a deficiency of Energy, Blood, Yin, or Yang. Herbal prescriptions can be given to remedy one or all of these. A celebrated energy tonic is Si Jun Zi Tang (four gentlemen decoction), which contains ginseng.

ANXIETY

An emotional and physiological state, anxiety encompasses feelings of unease, fear, and apprehension, and symptoms such as increased heartbeat, palpitations, clammy skin, disturbed sleep and appetite, muscle tension, inability to relax, restlessness, and digestive problems. In some people, the physical symptoms of anxiety can be severe enough to mimic a heart attack, with chest pains, breathlessness, pallor, and sweating.

Some anxious feelings are normal—before an exam or public speech, for example—and they serve to improve performance. It is only when anxiety starts to disrupt normal everyday activities that it becomes a problem. Anxiety can be caused by a personal, social, or physical problem such as a failing marriage, financial concerns, or illness.

A doctor may recommend counseling or psychotherapy to help with anxiety. In serious cases, an antianxiety drug might be prescribed for short periods. Herbs, Bach flower remedies, aromatherapy, relaxation, and acupuncture may all be helpful.

Herbalism

Herbs that relax and sedate the nervous system are good for anxiety. Chamomile is a gentle, calming herb—an infusion is especially recommended for children. Wood betony and wild oats strengthen the nervous system, cramp bark relaxes muscles, and lavender is an all-around relaxant. Other useful herbs are hops, valerian, motherwort, and passionflower (avoid high doses of passionflower during pregnancy, and avoid hops if you suffer from depression). Prepare these herbs as infusions or decoctions (decoctions are used when the herb is hard or woody). Vervain may be recommended by an herbalist.

THE CHILD'S POSE
Kneel on a soft surface and let your head sink toward the floor, resting your arms loosely by your sides, palms facing up. This pose relieves fatigue due to stress or anxiety.

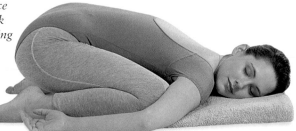

Bach flower remedies
Try taking rock rose for acute anxiety; mimulus for anxiety that is associated with illness, accidents and everyday life; aspen for anxiety with a sense of impending doom; and red chestnut for feelings of anxiety about other people.

Aromatherapy
One of the most widely used and versatile essential oils is lavender. It helps reduce tension and can be used in massage, a compress, or a bath, or its vapors can be inhaled from a bowl of hot water. Bergamot, marjoram, chamomile, cedarwood, cypress, frankincense, geranium, hyssop, jasmine, juniper, melissa, neroli, patchouli, rose, sandalwood, verbena, and ylang-ylang essential oils can all be used in the same ways.

Relaxation
Many problems seem far less insurmountable when viewed calmly. Relaxation and deep breathing (see page 114) may help you keep your problems in perspective.

Acupuncture
Anxiety is thought to derive from several different deficiencies. Points on the arms, legs, and trunk may be used to remedy the deficiency and balance the body.

STRESS
Although difficult to define, stress can be anything that disturbs a person's sense of well-being. What might be stressful for one person may be an enjoyable challenge for another. There are events, however, that nearly everyone considers to be stressful—divorce or separation, bereavement, moving, serious injury or illness, and job loss.

The body naturally responds to a stressful event by producing extra adrenaline. This increases the heart rate and blood flow to the muscles and slows down other processes, such as digestion, so that we are equipped to run or fight if necessary—the fight-or-flight response. Although most stressful events are unlikely to necessitate such a severe response, the body responds automatically in this age-old way.

The way we respond to stress—not so much the stress itself—determines whether the impact will be large or small. Coping poorly by turning to alcohol or ignoring the stressor usually makes the situation worse.

Over time, unrelieved stress may lead to anxiety, insomnia, and depression, or physical symptoms such as headaches, fatigue, or pains in the abdomen or back. Chronic stress is also considered a risk factor for serious illnesses such as hypertension and heart disease (see page 100) and should be taken very seriously.

Conventional medicine now embraces a wide range of natural therapies to manage stress, including relaxation techniques, creative visualization, biofeedback, and psychological counseling. Specific emotional and physical symptoms may be treated temporarily with medication, such as antianxiety drugs and muscle relaxants, but these are short-term remedies that merely deal with the symptoms of stress.

If you are under a great deal of stress, it's important to find the time to relax and unwind. Meditation is an effective stress reliever because it helps you achieve a deep sense of inner calm; massage and exercise can help by reducing muscle tension. Acupuncture can also be useful.

Meditation
Techniques for meditation are widely taught. There are various ways to meditate, but focusing on words (mantras or chants), breathing, or images are common in most types of meditation. See page 115 for a simple meditation exercise.

Massage
You can consult a massage therapist for a routine tailored to your particular needs, or you can practice simple massage techniques on yourself, your friends, and your family (see page 39). Massage helps muscles relax and relieves tension and pain by increasing the circulation of blood to the muscles.

Exercise
An excellent way of reducing tension due to stress and improving sleep quality is to get at least 20 minutes of aerobic exercise three times a week. Walking briskly, jogging, swimming, playing tennis, or cycling are all good forms of exercise that discharge tension and reduce levels of stress-related hormones in the body. Yoga (see page 43) and tai chi are other movement-based therapies that can help relieve the symptoms of stress. To achieve the best results, learn yoga and tai chi from a qualified teacher.

Acupuncture
By helping energy to flow freely around the body, acupuncture can be a great stress-reliever. Stress is believed to result either from Liver energy getting stuck or from the mind becoming unsettled.

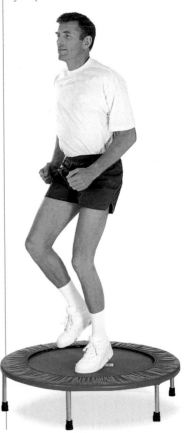

STRESS-RELIEVING EXERCISE
Any noncompetitive form of exercise can ease tension and help you feel more relaxed.

Relaxation

Some activities, such as listening to music, reading, and gardening, you can do on your own to unwind. With practice, other stress reducers like deep abdominal breathing and meditation are easily mastered.

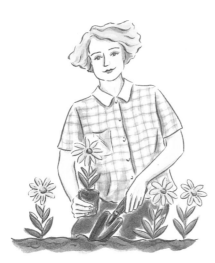

RELAXING PASTIMES
Sometimes a noncompetitive occupation such as gardening can be as therapeutic as yoga in relieving the mind and body of stress.

Breathing exercises help keep you calm when you're in a stressful situation. For instance, if you are sitting in a traffic jam or about to ask the boss for a raise, take one deep, slow breath in, then breathe out very slowly, relaxing as you do so.

Deep muscle relaxation

It is possible to moderate feelings of tension and alleviate your body's reaction to stress simply by lying down, closing your eyes, tuning out external noises, and allowing all your muscles to relax.

Lie flat on the floor with a blanket, towel, or small pillow under your head and neck for support. Let your arms fall out, palms up, about a foot away from your body, and let your legs fall slightly apart.

Close your eyes (putting something such as a towel over them can help you relax even more) and take a deep breath. As you inhale, tighten all the muscles in your body as much as you can, then, as you breathe out, allow them to relax completely. Repeat this twice, taking a few normal breaths in between deep breaths.

DEEP ABDOMINAL BREATHING

To practice deep abdominal breathing, set aside at least 10 minutes and find a warm place where you can lie down without being disturbed. Place a rolled blanket or towel under your head and neck, and let your legs relax. Close your eyes, place one hand on your chest and the other on your abdomen, and concentrate on the rhythm of your breathing. Inhale deeply into your abdomen and then breathe out slowly.

As you feel the rhythm of your breathing slow, start consciously to pull in your abdominal muscles when you exhale. Note which of your hands is moving when you breathe in and out—it should be the hand on your abdomen. When you feel that you are breathing into your abdomen, place your hands by your sides with the palms facing up.

Continue breathing in and out, concentrating only on your breath and the movement of your abdomen, but do not fall asleep. Remain in this position for 5 to 10 minutes.

BREATHING PRACTICE
Resting your hands on your abdomen and chest, feel them move in and out as you breathe. If your chest expands more than your abdomen, you are not breathing deeply enough.

Keep your head and neck supported with a rolled towel or blanket.

Essential oils heated in an oil burner can enhance deep relaxation.

PROGRESSIVE MUSCLE RELAXATION

The theory behind deep muscle relaxation is that before you can relax your body, you need to learn how your muscles feel when they are contracted and tense.

Progressive muscle relaxation is similar in principle to deep muscle relaxation, but instead of tensing all the muscles in your body simultaneously, you concentrate on tensing and relaxing one muscle group at a time. This can be done standing up or lying down, although you are more likely to achieve a state of deep relaxation lying down.

To practice deep muscle relaxation, tense the muscles in a specific muscle group for a count of 10. Then very slowly relax them. Breathe calmly and smoothly through your nose. Now move on to the next muscle group. When you have tensed and relaxed every part of your body, breathe deeply for about 10 minutes.

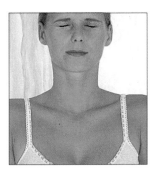

FOREHEAD AND EYES
Close your eyes tightly and tense the muscles in your forehead to form a deep frown. Then relax.

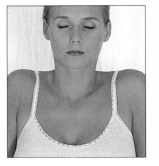

SHOULDERS
Hunch your shoulders, bringing them up toward your ears. Tense your neck. Then relax.

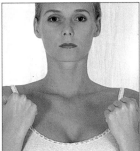

HANDS AND ARMS
Make your hands into fists and pull them in toward your shoulders. Then relax.

RELAXING THE MUSCLE GROUPS

By consciously contracting your muscles, holding them tensed for a few seconds, and then releasing them, you can systematically relax your entire body. Start with your hands and forearms, and work through all your muscles.

▶ *Hands and forearms—clench the fists, then let go*

▶ *Upper arms—clench the fists and bring them against the shoulders, then let go*

▶ *Forehead—frown and relax*

▶ *Eyebrows—raise up and release*

▶ *Jaw—thrust forward and release*

▶ *Neck—press the chin in and release*

▶ *Shoulders—hunch and let go*

▶ *Stomach—tense and relax*

▶ *Buttocks—tense and relax*

▶ *Thighs—tense and relax*

▶ *Legs—tense and relax*

▶ *Feet—flex and release*

MEDITATION

Meditation has been part of religious practice in many cultures for centuries. It is only relatively recently that the therapeutic value of meditation has been acknowledged. If you are suffering from stress, your mind may have a tendency to dwell on worries, failures, and other negative thoughts. The aim of meditation is to clear the mind by concentrating on one thing to the exclusion of everything else.

One simple method of meditation is to focus on your breathing. Find a position that you can comfortably maintain for about 20 minutes. This can be sitting, standing, or lying down, although sitting is preferable, since standing may be too tiring and lying down may make it easy to fall asleep. Try sitting on a straight-backed chair, on the floor on a cushion, or with your back against a wall.

To practice meditation, breathe in and out and count 1 in your head. Repeat, and count 2, and so on up to 10. Then begin at 1 again. After three cycles of counting to 10, stop counting and focus on the sensations and movements of each breath—the up and down motion of your chest, the air going in and out of your nostrils, the texture of the air, and any other feelings that you are aware of. Focus only on the spot where you first feel the air hit your body. This may be the tip of your nose, the back of your nostrils, or your throat. Whenever thoughts intrude, gently bring your mind back to your breathing.

FOCUS ON YOUR BREATHING
Although it takes some practice, you should be able to clear your mind of everything except an awareness of the physical sensation of breathing.

Rest your hands in your lap and relax your shoulders and arms.

SPECIFIC PROBLEMS

Some emotions, such as grief, will affect everyone sometime. Other problems, such as eating disorders, may result from individual, deeply rooted pyschological problems.

You may not be able to surmount all emotional problems on your own, but with help most can be alleviated. If you feel you cannot cope on a day-to-day basis, it is important to seek psychological counseling or medical help. In addition, you may obtain some relief with homeopathic remedies, hypnotherapy, relaxation techniques, Bach flower remedies, or massage.

BEREAVEMENT

People who experience the death of a loved one need to come to terms with their loss. The process of grieving has various stages, ranging from anger to acceptance. In some cases the bereaved cannot progress from one stage to another, or become mired in depression that lasts beyond the normal grieving period. It is important to consult your doctor if these feelings persist.

You should also make the most of supportive family and friends, or contact a social worker, clergyman, self-help group, bereavement counselor, psychotherapist, or psychiatrist. A bereaved person should be encouraged to express grief and not suppress it. Prolonged use of tranquilizers and sedatives is no longer recommended because they can inhibit the natural grieving process. Homeopathy and counseling may be helpful alternatives.

Homeopathy
Arnica For shock and wanting to be left alone in the early stages of bereavement.
Aconite For feeling afraid and on the verge of collapse.
Opium For emotional numbness that is associated with grief.
Nux vomica For anger toward others in the late stages of bereavement.
Phosphoric acid For depression and feelings of apathy.
Ignatia For difficulty in controlling the emotions.

Counseling
Bereavement counseling is widely available —your doctor will be able to advise you. Clergymen and laypeople are also trained to counsel the bereaved and are usually able to visit people in their own homes.

EMOTIONAL TRAUMA
Severe emotional shock, or trauma, can be caused by a frightening or tragic event, such as a serious car accident or a mugging. Emotional trauma causes an extreme reaction in the mind and body; initial denial or emotional numbness gives way to feelings of anxiety, panic, or depression that can cause rapid breathing, hyperventilation, palpitations, churning stomach, pallor, and cold, clammy sweating.

Conventionally, doctors will treat severe emotional trauma with counseling and, in extreme cases, tranquilizers or antidepressants. Of the natural therapies, the most useful include acupressure, homeopathy, and Bach flower remedies.

Acupressure
If someone faints from emotional trauma, they should be put in the recovery position and pressure should be applied upward on point GV 26 (see page 76). This is located two-thirds of the way up between your upper lip and your nose.

Homeopathy
Aconite For sudden shock, terror, or panic and palpitations.
Arnica For acute shock, particularly after an accident.
Ignatia For hysteria.
Coffea For emotional shock and insomnia due to a racing mind.

Bach flower remedies
Rescue remedy, the primary treatment for shock and trauma, is a special mixture of Bach flower remedies that can be taken in an emergency. Rock rose can be used for severe

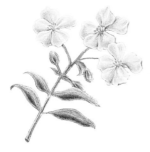

ROCK ROSE
This Bach flower remedy is recommended for treating feelings of shock, fear, or panic.

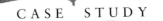
A Panic Attack Sufferer

Short-lived episodes in which the sufferer feels breathless and experiences palpitations, dizziness, sweating, trembling, and a fear of fainting or asphyxiating are frightening. These symptoms may be triggered by specific incidents or may stem from a general sense of deep anxiety. Identifying the cause of panic attacks is the first step to overcoming them.

Louise is 27. Three months ago she got a job as a translator in a large city over 200 miles from her home. This meant moving away from her family and living in an apartment. In the past, she has suffered from insomnia and anxiety, and has taken sleeping pills.

Now that Louise is living alone in a new city, her anxiety is returning. When traveling to work in the morning she feels that she cannot control her breathing and she is frightened of fainting. The more she worries about her anxiety attacks, the worse she seems to feel. Recently the attacks have worsened and she experiences breathlessness, palpitations, and dizziness, especially on the crowded commuter trains that she must take to work.

WHAT LOUISE SHOULD DO

Louise has to take some action to stop her symptoms escalating and help her regain control. To start, she should learn some basic relaxation and breathing techniques, which she can practice during an attack. She could also try taking a homeopathic or a Bach flower remedy for her symptoms.

Louise also needs to look at the reasons for her anxiety and find ways to overcome them. Practical measures include getting involved in more social activities so that she does not feel so isolated; moving into an apartment where she can share with another person rather than living alone; and—at least on a short-term basis—traveling to work before rush hour.

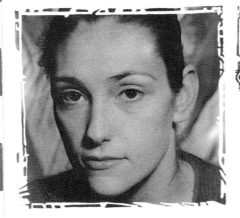

HEALTH
If left untreated, past anxiety or depressive episodes can predispose you to future health problems.

WORK
Going to work in a new and unfamiliar environment is a potentially stressful experience and can cause anxiety or even depression in susceptible people.

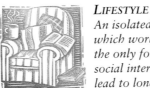

LIFESTYLE
An isolated lifestyle in which work provides the only form of social interaction can lead to loneliness and depression, which may then manifest themselves as anxiety and panic attacks.

Action Plan

HEALTH
Make an appointment with a homeopath and follow the recommended treatment for as long as necessary. Try taking a Bach flower remedy; also learn breathing and relaxation techniques.

WORK
Leave for work early in the morning to avoid crowded highways and public transportation.

LIFESTYLE
Join a local club or service group to expand social life. Place an ad in the newspaper for a room in a shared apartment or house.

HOW THINGS TURNED OUT FOR LOUISE

Rather than looking to home for support, Louise decided to become involved in her new community. She now attends weekly yoga classes in a gym near her workplace. This has helped her to feel more relaxed and her anxiety attacks are far less frequent. A message left on the bulletin board at work resulted in some apartment-sharing possibilities and several new acquaintances. She also takes the homeopathic remedy *Gelsemium* for panic attacks.

Controlling panic attacks

When you hyperventilate you take in too much oxygen. Inhaling your own carbon dioxide from a paper bag will compensate for this. If you begin to hyperventilate during a panic attack, try to relax by breathing deeply and slowly.

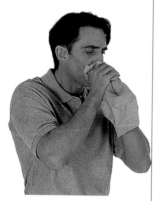

BREATHING INTO A BAG
The paper bag should make a seal over your mouth and nose. Inhale and exhale as calmly and slowly as you can.

shock, and star-of-Bethlehem is recommended for shock after being told serious news.

PANIC ATTACKS

A panic attack is usually the result of extreme anxiety or a phobia (see page 120). It is a brief attack of intense fear. Often panic attacks are associated with certain places such as crowded stores, elevators, or heights. Physical symptoms include hyperventilation, a sensation of not being able to breathe, palpitations, dizziness, chest pains, sweating, trembling, and hot or cold flashes. Although frightening and unpleasant, panic attacks are not dangerous.

Behavioral therapy, tranquilizers, antidepressants, and relaxation might be recommended by a doctor to treat panic attacks. Any underlying anxieties will also be addressed. Of the natural remedies, Bach flower remedies, homeopathy, and relaxation may help.

Bach flower remedies

The Bach flower remedy rock rose is useful at times of extreme terror and panic.

Homeopathy

Aconite For panic attacks and feelings of intense anxiety.

Gelsemium For trembling, palpitations, and feelings of anxiety.

Relaxation

Deep breathing and relaxation methods (see page 99 and pages 114–115) may help prevent panic attacks or lessen their severity.

DEPRESSION

The symptoms of depression include crying spells, despair, sadness, difficulty sleeping, reduced appetite, apathy, irritability, and lack of interest in sex. Most people have short periods of these feelings that are a natural response to specific events such as divorce or job loss. For others, depression can occur for no apparent reason and it can become chronic. In severe depression, there may be suicidal thoughts, and feelings of intense guilt and worthlessness.

Depression may have a physical cause. Some women become depressed after giving birth, and some people experience depression in the winter because of a reduction in the number of daylight hours (seasonal affective disorder, or SAD). A viral infection or an underactive thyroid gland can also cause feelings of depression. Seek medical advice if depression persists or is severe.

In orthodox medicine, the most common treatment for depression is a short course of antidepressant drugs. Group or individual psychotherapy may also be recommended, and electroconvulsive therapy (ECT) is still used in many hospitals for severe chronic depression. There is also a range of natural remedies that may help.

Herbalism

Wild oats have antidepressant properties and can strengthen the nervous system. Ginseng may also strengthen the nervous system and promote a sense of well-being (avoid if you suffer from hypertension). Lemon balm, rosemary, and basil may all have antidepressant properties (avoid rosemary during pregnancy). Numerous clinical trials have demonstrated that St. John's wort brings symptomatic relief in various forms of mild depression and is considered to work as effectively as some synthetic drugs. All these herbs can be taken as decoctions or infusions.

Bach flower remedies

Mustard is recommended for gloom and despair; sweet chestnut for great anguish and morbidity; and willow for depression and bitterness. Other useful remedies are gorse for hopelessness; larch for despair and lack of confidence; pine for blame and guilt; and elm for depression with anxiety.

Massage

A massage using essential oils diluted with a base oil can lift your spirits. Essential oils thought to have an uplifting effect include bergamot, orange, lemon balm, jasmine, neroli, or rose. Massage alone may help, too.

Exercise

Moderate exercise causes the release of endorphins and enkephalins into the bloodstream. These are natural substances that promote a feeling of well-being and can alleviate lethargy and depression. Try to swim, walk, or jog every day.

Chinese herbalism

Depression is considered to be due to one of about 10 disharmonies, but the most common are Liver Energy stagnation and Heart Yin deficiency. Consult a Chinese herbalist for an individual prescription.

Naturopathy

Avoid alcohol, dairy products, coffee and tea, smoking, processed foods, red meat, eggs, refined sugar, and flour. Eat plenty of fresh green vegetables, fruits, whole grains, peas, and beans. Tryptophan is a naturally occurring antidepressant found in poultry, fish, peas, beans, peanut butter, and nuts. Take vitamin B complex, brewer's yeast, or a multivitamin and mineral supplement.

Counseling

Talking to a professional counselor can help you sort out personal issues that may be contributing to your depression. You can discuss problems about work, relationships, alcohol, drugs, and money—anything that is troubling you.

A counselor will encourage you to reveal your experiences and feelings, which are then discussed to gain insight into your depression. Counseling is often carried out on a one-to-one basis, although sometimes couple or family counseling is recommended.

Psychotherapy is also useful. It's more intensive and prolonged than counseling—between six months and two years (or longer) as opposed to a few weeks. It focuses on your past experiences and relationships, the impact they have had on your life, and how they may influence your current responses and behavior patterns.

ADDICTION

People can become addicted to legal substances such as nicotine, alcohol, and caffeine; illegal drugs such as cocaine and heroin; and prescription drugs such as tranquilizers. Certain activities like gambling or shopping, if carried to extremes, are also considered to be addictions.

Drug addiction can be either physical or psychological, or both. If psychologically dependent, you will experience cravings and distress when the drug is withdrawn. If you are physically dependent, in addition to psychological symptoms, withdrawal will cause shaking and trembling, insomnia, sweating, a rapid heartbeat, and, occasionally, convulsions.

There are withdrawal programs in larger hospitals, special drug rehabilitation centers, and clinics for help and counseling. Sometimes a less harmful drug is given temporarily to substitute for the drug that is being withdrawn, for example, methadone to replace heroin.

Acupuncture and naturopathy may be useful in relieving the symptoms of withdrawal. Hypnotherapy and counseling can help you gain control over undesired behavior.

Acupuncture

Both physical and mental withdrawal symptoms may be treated with acupuncture. Ear acupuncture is thought by some to stimulate the brain to produce more of its own calming chemicals. Tiny ear stud needles may be put in place for the person to press himself between treatments. Traditional Chinese acupuncture can be used to treat a body weakened by drugs.

Naturopathy

To cleanse your system, naturopaths recommend three days of light fasting. During this time you may eat fruit and drink vegetable and fruit juices. This sort of diet should be attempted only under the supervision of a doctor or naturopath.

After a period of fasting, it is important to take vitamin B complex, brewer's yeast, or a multivitamin and mineral supplement —even addictions to coffee and nicotine can deplete the body of essential nutrients. A healthful diet that consists of fresh fruits and vegetables, whole grains, and legumes should be followed.

Hypnotherapy

A hypnotherapist will help you change your behavior regarding the addictive substance, perhaps by reminding you of its undesirable qualities, or by helping you discover the underlying cause of your addiction. Although most people can be hypnotized to some degree, not everyone responds to hypnotherapy. You must be able to relax and trust your hypnotherapist. Some people feel more comfortable with a therapist of the same sex.

Counseling

One-to-one or group counseling can help identify the underlying reasons for the addiction and provide emotional support during the withdrawal period.

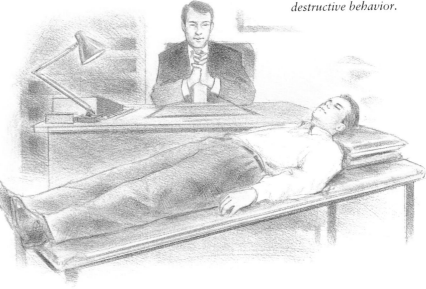

HYPNOTHERAPY
To help you overcome your addiction, the therapist will put you in a trance and make suggestions to help you control your destructive behavior.

EATING DISORDERS

Anorexia nervosa, bulimia, and compulsive eating are all serious eating disorders. Sufferers may either be underweight or overweight, but they are all victims of abnormal eating patterns.

Anorexia is characterized by severe weight loss due to self-starvation; usually the sufferer has a distorted body image and a fear of becoming fat. Bulimia involves bingeing, followed by purging through self-induced vomiting or laxative abuse. Like anorexics, bulimics fear being fat.

Compulsive eating is defined as uncontrolled and chronic bouts of overeating that in some cases lead to obesity. Psychological problems can cause compulsive eating, and these problems can be exacerbated by the ensuing weight gain.

Treatment of eating disorders involves getting sufferers to acknowledge the problem, followed by medical supervision of eating habits. People with severe anorexia may be hospitalized to allow strict control of their diets, and may be given antidepressants.

Psychologists see unusual eating habits as indicative of a poor self-image and low self-esteem. Any therapy that increases positive feelings is helpful.

Relaxation

People with eating disorders usually have deep-rooted psychological problems that may be exacerbated by stress. Relaxation may ease tension and increase feelings of well-being. Practicing yoga, deep breathing, or other relaxation techniques can help.

Hypnotherapy

It is thought that a suggestion given under hypnosis may help change a person's attitudes toward food. Hypnosis may also be a useful therapy for discovering unconscious anxieties and finding ways to express them in a less harmful way.

Chinese medicine

Practitioners of Chinese medicine view eating disorders as a weakness of the digestive system and the Spleen. Acupuncture and Chinese herbs are used to tone the digestive system and to enable the stomach to digest and absorb food more easily.

Counseling

By helping you get in touch with underlying emotional problems, counseling can help you understand the reasons for your eating disorder. Counseling can take the form of one-to-one or group therapy sessions. Emotional support is essential for people trying to recover from eating disorders.

PHOBIAS

A persistent, irrational fear of something is known as a phobia. Typical phobias include a fear of open spaces (agoraphobia), a fear of enclosed spaces (claustrophobia), and a fear of spiders (arachnophobia). When confronted with a feared activity, situation, or object, the phobic person may experience intense anxiety or a panic attack. Although some 20 percent of the population is affected by simple phobias, such as a fear of dogs, cats, or spiders, some phobias can be disabling. For instance, agoraphobia may cause the sufferer to become housebound.

Psychologists suggest that phobias are learned responses, since people with phobias have often been brought up by someone with a similar fear. A frightening experience, particularly in childhood, can also lead to a phobia.

A common treatment for phobias is behavioral therapy, but antidepressants may also be prescribed for agoraphobia. Relaxation, homeopathy, and hypnotherapy may help.

Relaxation

Controlling your breathing (see page 99) has a calming effect.

Homeopathy

Phosphorus For fear of the dark.
Gelsemium For fright.
Lycopodium For great apprehension.
Sulfur For fear of heights with giddiness.

Hypnotherapy

A hypnotherapist will place you in a trance and suggest that you are calm, relaxed, and no longer frightened of the object of your phobia. You may be taught self-hypnosis techniques to reinforce the treatment.

ARACHNOPHOBIA
Although some people feel uncomfortable when they are near a spider, an arachnophobe experiences an intense, uncontrollable fear even when looking at a picture of a spider.

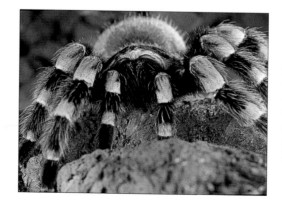

CHAPTER 9

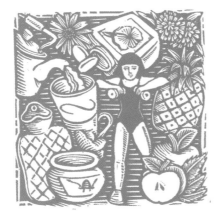

WOMEN'S HEALTH

*Most women, at least once in their lives,
will suffer from a disorder or complaint that falls
under the all-encompassing term "women's problems."
This may be premenstrual syndrome (PMS), painful
periods, yeast infection, or something more serious such
as pelvic inflammatory disease (PID). If the problem
is chronic—as PMS is for many women—natural
remedies such as acupressure and relaxation
can be extremely helpful and eliminate the
need for conventional drugs.*

GYNECOLOGICAL PROBLEMS

Some of the symptoms of female problems, whether menstrual, pregnancy related, or menopausal, can be dealt with in simple, natural ways. There is no need to suffer.

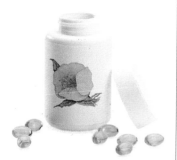

EVENING PRIMROSE OIL
One 500-milligram capsule of evening primrose oil, taken every day for at least three months, may help to ease PMS symptoms.

Many gynecological disorders are taken for granted as part of a woman's biological inheritance. Some, like premenstrual syndrome, do not necessarily need medical attention, but certain natural remedies may bring relief.

PREMENSTRUAL SYNDROME (PMS)

It is common during the two weeks before menstruation for women to experience symptoms of PMS such as irritability, depression, mood swings, breast tenderness, fatigue, food cravings, headaches, digestive problems, and fluid retention. The causes of PMS are unclear, but diet, stress, and hormonal changes have been implicated.

Some women are prescribed the contraceptive pill to minimize hormonal fluctuations; herbalism, relaxation, exercise, naturopathy, and acupuncture are natural alternatives.

Herbalism

An infusion of dandelion leaves can be taken for water retention, and an infusion of raspberry and chamomile for cramping pains. Evening primrose oil capsules may help relieve PMS symptoms, particularly tender swollen breasts.

Relaxation

Stress and fatigue may exacerbate the symptoms of PMS, and relaxation may bring relief. For best results, practice every day for 20 to 30 minutes. Yoga (see page 110) or meditation (see page 114) is effective.

Exercise

Regular aerobic exercise in which your target heart rate (see page 101) is maintained for 20 minutes or more may relieve the symptoms of PMS by releasing pain-relieving endorphins into the bloodstream. Endorphins also lift your mood and promote relaxation. Stepping up your exercise program during the two weeks before your period may help to prevent some symptoms.

Naturopathy

Try taking the following supplements: 300 milligrams of magnesium a day, 400 units of vitamin E, or 50 milligrams of vitamin B_6 (consult a doctor about vitamin E if you have hypertension or heart disease). Take the supplements for at least three months to assess their effectiveness. If you are prone to bloating, cut down on salty and refined foods.

FEMALE PELVIC ORGANS

The uterus lies behind the bladder. It is lined with specialized tissue, called the endometrium, which thickens each month and is shed during menstruation.

THE MENSTRUAL CYCLE
Each month an egg, or ovum, is released from one of two ovaries and moves down a fallopian tube. If the ovum is not fertilized, it enters the uterus and leaves the body via the vagina during menstruation.

An ovary produces eggs, estrogen, and progesterone.

A fallopian tube is situated on either side of the uterus.

The uterus has a thick outer wall of muscle.

Bladder

The vagina joins the uterus and the vulva.

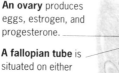

DID YOU KNOW?
It is estimated that approximately 85 to 95 percent of menstruating women in the United States suffer from PMS at one time or another. Most women rely on self-help measures for symptom relief.

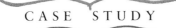
A PMS Sufferer

Some women report personality changes and disrupted home lives due to hormonal changes prior to menstruation. Children, partners, and friends may bear the brunt of a woman's PMS-related mood swings, and her work or studies may be affected through loss of concentration due to fatigue, depression, or anxiety.

Emily is 30 and has two children. When her younger child, Amanda, aged six, started school a year ago, Emily went back to work as a legal secretary. Although she enjoys her job, she is severely affected by PMS every month, which worries her because she knows she is less efficient then. She becomes depressed, tired, and tearful; loses confidence in herself; and suffers from outbursts of anger directed at her husband and children. Recently, she was taken aback when she lost her temper and slapped Amanda hard several times for minor misbehavior.

Emily had PMS before Amanda was born but was fine for a couple of years after her birth. The problem has become significantly worse since she returned to work.

WHAT EMILY SHOULD DO

Emily needs to assess why her PMS has become worse since she went back to work, and whether she is overextending herself. By keeping a menstrual diary she can keep track of symptoms and may find that they coincide with a busy time at work, or are worse when there are problems at home, such as when her children are sick.

Emily should also look at her diet for clues to changes in her behavior. She may be eating foods, particularly in the week before her period, that trigger or exacerbate her symptoms.

Most important, Emily should think about the ways she can reduce her stress levels, both at work and at home. Acupuncture may help.

Action Plan

STRESS
Take more time to relax. Get help with the housework and ask a friend to look after the children after work when symptoms are at their worst.

DIET
Cut down on caffeine. Add less salt to food in cooking and at the table. Take vitamin supplements.

HEALTH
Make an appointment to see an acupuncturist and consider a course of treatment. Go swimming with the children a couple of times a week and walk as much as possible.

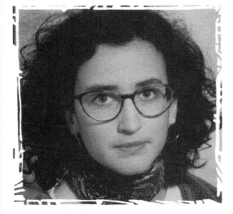

STRESS
Many women's premenstrual symptoms are worse when they are tired or tense.

DIET
A high-salt intake can encourage water retention, and a high-sugar diet may cause mood swings. Caffeine exacerbates the symptoms of PMS, as does a lack of exercise.

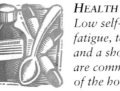

HEALTH
Low self-esteem, fatigue, tearfulness, and a short temper are common effects of the hormonal changes in the days before menstruation.

HOW THINGS TURNED OUT FOR EMILY

Emily has started to pay more attention to her diet and has begun a regular exercise routine, swimming twice a week and walking home from work. For three months she visited an acupuncturist, but she lost the impetus to continue when her symptoms improved.

Despite this improvement Emily's premenstrual symptoms vary from month to month, but she is more lenient now, allowing herself more time for relaxation.

Acupressure for painful periods

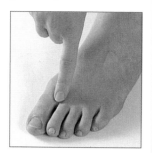

PRESSURE POINT LIV 2 This is located at the junction between the big toe and the second toe.

THE NORMAL MENSTRUAL CYCLE Regular ovulation and menstruation depend upon the rise and fall of the female hormones, estrogen and progesterone. Ovulation usually occurs on the 14th day of the cycle—just after estrogen peaks. Menstruation occurs when the levels of both hormones drop. If hormone production becomes erratic, periods become irregular.

Many women find that their premenstrual symptoms are aggravated by alcohol and caffeine, so it's best to avoid beer, wine, and spirits, in addition to cola, coffee, and tea. A drop in blood sugar, which can produce symptoms, may be prevented by eating small meals at regular intervals instead of three large meals. It is also important to eat plenty of fiber-rich foods such as vegetables, fruits, and bran to avoid constipation.

Acupuncture
PMS may respond well to acupuncture, which can ease the emotional as well as the physical symptoms.

PAINFUL PERIODS (DYSMENORRHEA)
There are two types of menstrual pain. Primary dysmenorrhea, caused by the muscular contractions of the uterus, is experienced as menstrual cramps during the first two or three days of menstruation. It is common in teenage girls and young women.

Secondary dysmenorrhea occurs when periods suddenly become painful. This is usually due to an underlying condition such as fibroids or endometriosis.

Conventionally, primary dysmenorrhea is treated with painkillers, the contraceptive pill, or drugs that inhibit the production of prostaglandins—hormones that can cause uterine cramping. For secondary dysmenorrhea, the underlying cause is treated.

A variety of alternative therapies may be effective for easing the cramps of primary dysmenorrhea. These include acupressure, homeopathy, yoga, and transcutaneous electrical nerve stimulation (TENS). If you think you have secondary dysmenorrhea you should seek medical treatment for the underlying condition.

Acupressure
Apply pressure to points Liv 2, Liv 3 (see page 131) and Sp 6 (see page 128). Liv 3 is found two finger widths toward the ankle from the junction of the big and second toes. You can find point Sp 6 just off the edge of the shinbone, three finger widths above the inner ankle. Ankle bands that continuously stimulate this point are also available.

Homeopathy
Colocynth For cramps eased by pressure.
Sepia For a sensation of heaviness and bearing down, irritability, and tiredness.
Chamomilla For pains that come and go and resemble labor pains.

Yoga
Recurrent menstrual pain may be eased by practicing yoga regularly. Breathing exercises and a movement called the cobra (see page 99) can be especially helpful.

Transcutaneous electrical nerve stimulation (TENS)
Menstrual pain usually responds well to the application of minute electrical impulses to the affected nerves. Applied by means of a portable transmitter, TENS is thought to work by blocking pain signals to the brain and stimulating the release of natural painkillers called endorphins.

Although TENS may relieve immediate pain, acupuncture may be a more appropriate therapy for relieving long-term recurrent pain. A TENS machine may be available through a doctor or physiotherapy clinic.

IRREGULAR MENSTRUATION
Periods that are unpredictable in frequency, do not follow the usual 22- to 35-day cycle, or vary in the amount of bleeding are termed irregular. Irregular menstruation is normal at puberty and at the menopause, but at other times it may be a symptom of another problem such as a hormonal disturbance, eating disorder, or stress.

Conventional treatment depends very much on the cause of irregular bleeding. It is important that you see your doctor or gynecologist for a diagnosis before turning to natural therapies such as herbalism. Often, doctors will treat hormonal imbalances with drugs that normalize the cycle.

Herbalism
If your periods fluctuate in the months or years leading up to your menopause, chaste tree may help by acting on the pituitary gland to normalize hormonal levels. False unicorn

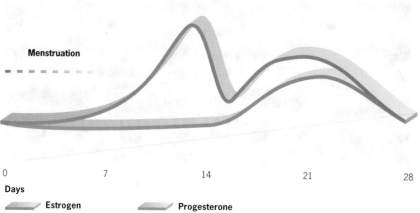

Menstruation

Days

Estrogen   Progesterone

root can help to stimulate ovarian hormones and may be useful in regulating periods after the prolonged use of oral contraceptives.

ABSENCE OF MENSTRUATION (AMENORRHEA)

Menstrual periods stop naturally during pregnancy and menopause. You should be concerned, however, if your periods stop at other times. It is not uncommon for women to miss one or even two menstrual periods, but if your amenorrhea has no obvious cause and lasts longer than a few months, you should seek medical help. The same applies to girls who have not begun to menstruate by the age of 16. Amenorrhea can be caused by a multitude of factors, including physical abnormalities, chronic disease, hormonal imbalance, and malnutrition.

Conventional treatment addresses the underlying cause. Homeopathy, herbalism, and naturopathy may also help to restore a healthy menstrual cycle, but it is important to see your doctor for a diagnosis before starting these treatments.

Homeopathy

Pulsatilla For periods that are delayed, irregular, or absent, especially at puberty.
Sepia For amenorrhea accompanied by depression and wanting to be alone.
Aconite For periods that stop after a shock.
Ignatia For periods that cease due to grief.

Herbalism

If you miss periods after discontinuing the contraceptive pill, an infusion of black cohosh may help. Do not use this herb if you suspect that you may be pregnant.

Naturopathy

Overexercising or very limited calorie intake may inhibit the menstrual cycle. Sudden or extreme losses in body fat cause the body to shut down certain systems. One theory holds that the body naturally stops a malnourished woman from becoming pregnant, because she does not have enough stored energy to support a developing baby.

A deficiency of zinc can lead to amenorrhea, so increasing the amount of fish, cheese, lean meat, and poultry in your diet may help. Vegetarians, breast-feeding women, and pubescent girls, in particular, may be more deficient in zinc than other women. Supplements may be advisable, but consult your doctor before taking them.

Vitamin B_6 may also help in certain cases of amenorrhea, but if you want to take a supplement, take a vitamin B complex to ensure that you include all the B vitamins rather than limiting yourself to only one. Natural sources of vitamin B_6 are wheat germ, bananas, potatoes, and poultry. Your vitamin B intake should increase as your protein intake increases.

VAGINAL DISCHARGE

Some vaginal discharge is a natural part of the menstrual cycle. The amount of discharge depends on the individual and where she is in her menstrual cycle. Discharge needs to be treated only if it is profuse, smelly, thick, green, yellow, or associated with vaginal soreness, itching, or bleeding.

An unusual vaginal discharge is often caused by an infection, such as a yeast infection, or a sexually transmitted disease. A tampon left in the vagina too long may also cause a discharge.

Conventional treatment consists of identifying the cause of the discharge and treating any infection, for example, giving antifungal suppositories and creams for a yeast infection.

Natural remedies including naturopathy, homeopathy, herbalism, or Chinese herbalism can be used in conjunction with whatever your doctor has prescribed to ease the symptoms of vaginal discharge.

Naturopathy

If vaginal discharge is caused by a yeast infection, naturopaths say that it may be made worse by consuming sugary foods and foods containing yeast, such as bread.

Plain, live-culture yogurt inserted into the vagina three times a day with an applicator may improve the bacterial environment. A large clove of garlic wrapped in sterile gauze attached to a piece of cotton and placed high in the vagina may also help (remove and replace the cotton and garlic twice a day). If

continued on page 128

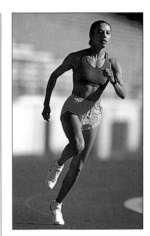

OVEREXERCISING
Extreme physical exercise can disrupt the menstrual cycle by reducing a woman's body fat level. Running is the sport most often associated with athletic or exercise-induced amenorrhea.

VITAMIN B_6 AND AMENORRHEA
Boost your dietary intake of vitamin B_6 with poultry, potatoes, wheat germ, bananas, raisins, and sunflower seeds.

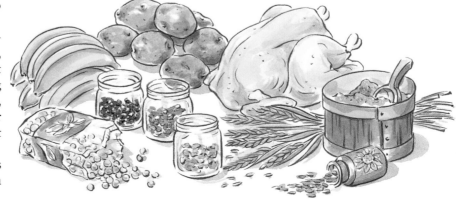

The Homeopath

Following a system of medicine that aims to cure illness by treating the underlying cause, a homeopath will look at the physical symptoms and emotional state of a patient with menstrual problems and choose an appropriate remedy.

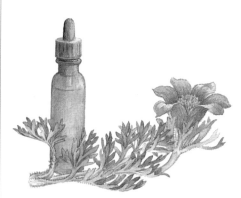

WINDFLOWER
Homeopaths use very dilute substances to treat illnesses. The remedy that is derived from windflower—Pulsatilla—is used to treat amenorrhea and other menstrual problems.

A homeopath bears in mind that menstrual problems have many physical and emotional causes, from excessive weight loss or gain to deficiencies of pituitary or ovarian hormones to trauma and long-standing repression of emotions.

Prolonged use of the contraceptive pill may also be to blame. Birth control pills manipulate hormone levels, and after discontinuing the pills, temporary infertility may occur. Homeopathic treatment in this instance can sometimes help to restore the natural menstrual cycle that was interrupted.

Who practices homeopathy?
Most states allow anyone who is a licensed health care professional to practice homeopathy. About half of the 3,000 recognized practitioners in the U.S. are physicians; others are naturopaths, chiropractors, dentists, and veterinarians. Nurses and physician assistants can also practice homeopathy, but only under the supervision of a medical doctor. For a nominal fee the National Center for Homeopathy will send you a list of practitioners in your area. The address is 801 North Fairfax Street, Alexandria, Virginia 22314.

What procedures are used when diagnosing the causes of menstrual problems?
Initially, the homeopath will obtain a complete medical history for you and your family, in order to evaluate inherited tendencies. The types of medication you have taken, past experiences, current lifestyle, mood and behavior patterns, and diet are also considered. The homeopath will also establish whether pregnancy, nursing, or menopause is the cause of absent, irregular, or heavy periods.

Will a homeopath work in conjunction with a doctor?
A patient may have visited a doctor first and found that conventional treatments have not helped. Alternatively, homeopathy may be the first choice of treatment. In either case, a good homeopath will encourage you to keep your doctor informed about homeopathic treatment. Sometimes, a homeopath will refer you to a conventional doctor for a checkup or diagnostic tests to exclude the possibility of serious underlying illness.

HOW TO TAKE HOMEOPATHIC REMEDIES

Remedies should be protected from contamination as much as possible. Do not handle them or take the pills directly after eating, smoking, or drinking beverages that contain alcohol or caffeine.

TAKING THE REMEDIES
Place a pill on a spoon and put it under your tongue. Avoid touching the pills with your fingers.

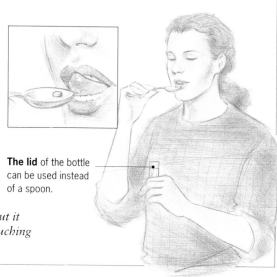

The lid of the bottle can be used instead of a spoon.

Which remedies are used to treat menstrual problems?

Homeopaths believe that treatment should be directed not only at the menstrual problem itself but also at the character and condition of the individual. As such, there is no single homeopathic remedy for a specific disorder—treatment is always individualized. Recommended and widely used remedies are:

Calcarea (made from oyster shells) For heavy periods and the emotional and physical symptoms of premenstrual tension.

Natrum muriaticum (made from sodium chloride) For late periods accompanied by headache.

Colocynthis (made from bitter cucumber) For menstrual pains with severe cramps that are relieved by warmth.

Aconite (made from monkshood) For absent periods following shock, fear, or a chill.

Pulsatilla (made from windflower) For period pain, irregular periods, and mood swings.

Dulcamara (made from bittersweet) For absent or irregular periods and a sensitivity to cold and damp. Menses are watery when they occur, and breasts are swollen and sore.

Kali carbonicum (made from potassium carbonate) For delayed or difficult first menses and for women who are overweight, exhausted, anxious, have difficulty swallowing, and leucorrhea—constant, heavy discharge—with laborlike pains.

Lycopodium (made from club moss) For absent periods with leucorrhea, vaginal dryness, and burning sensations that are worse during and after intercourse.

Magnesia phosphorica (made from magnesium phosphate) For menstrual cramps that are soothed by heat, pressure, and movement.

Sepia (made from cuttlefish ink) For a heavy, dull, or dragging sensation in the lower abdomen during menstruation. Also recommended for irritability and fatigue.

How soon should a remedy work?

In some cases, a single remedy may activate a cure. For many women, however, the menstrual cycle may be normalized after several consultations with the homeopath. When menstrual problems have several different causes, a sequence of remedies, individualized for the patient, may be required.

Dulcamara and many other remedies come in liquid form.

Club moss is used as the basis for *Lycopodium.*

Lycopodium pills are recommended for amenorrhea.

Monkshood is the raw material for the remedy *Aconite.*

HERBS AND HOMEOPATHY
Many homeopathic remedies are made from highly dilute extracts of common and exotic herbs.

Bittersweet is the basis of the remedy *Dulcamara.*

Take Aconite for periods missed due to shock.

127

Acupressure for endometriosis

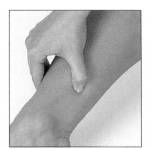

PRESSURE POINT SP 6
This is on the inside of the ankle, three finger widths up from the ankle bone, just off the edge of the shinbone.

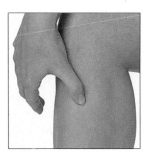

PRESSURE POINT ST 36
This point is located four finger widths below the kneecap toward the outside of the shinbone.

this causes irritation, remove it immediately. Eating garlic, especially raw garlic, may also help fight infection.

Homeopathy
Calcarea carbonica For a milky, yellow discharge accompanied by cold, damp hands and feet, a burning pain in the uterus, and unusual morning hunger.
Sepia For an offensive, yellowish green discharge that is worse before menstruating and associated with constipation.
Pulsatilla For any vaginal discharge, but especially one that is thick, milky, and burning, and is accompanied by mood swings and chills.

Herbalism
Make an infusion with two parts each of American cranesbill, bethroot (trillium), echinacea, and periwinkle, and one part cleavers. Use as a vaginal douche twice a day.

Chinese herbalism
Persistent vaginal discharge may respond to treatment with Chinese herbs. Consult a practitioner of Chinese medicine for an individual prescription.

ENDOMETRIOSIS
For reasons that remain unclear, parts of the uterine lining sometimes implant themselves on other parts of the body—usually other organs of the pelvic cavity. This condition is known as endometriosis. These uterine fragments respond to hormones by bleeding during menstruation, causing the formation of cysts or nodules.

This may result in heavier than normal periods, abdominal pain that is often worse at the end of the period, pain on intercourse, diarrhea, constipation, and, occasionally, infertility. However, in some cases, endometriosis can be symptomless.

Conventional diagnosis may involve investigation with a laparoscope (a small viewing instrument inserted into the abdominal cavity). Subsequent treatment may include the contraceptive pill or a similar drug, such as danazol, which prevents ovulation and bleeding. In certain cases, surgery may be required. Complementary therapies like acupressure and naturopathy will not cure the cause but may help to relieve the pain of endometriosis.

Acupressure
Apply steady pressure to points Sp 6 and point Liv 2 (see page 124). Liv 2 is located at the junction of the big and second toes

and may help with the pain associated with heavy menstruation. Stimulating pressure point St 36 is also useful for abdominal pains that are related to endometriosis.

Naturopathy
Eating foods such as oily fish and taking cod liver oil or other fish oil supplements is believed to inhibit the production of prostaglandins—the hormones that can cause uterine cramping—and may ease pain.

Supplements of vitamin B complex, calcium, magnesium, and up to 500 units of vitamin E per day to balance hormone levels may help. If you have high blood pressure or heart disease, consult a doctor before taking vitamin E supplements.

VAGINISMUS
Involuntary, painful spasms of the muscles at the entrance to the vagina are described as vaginismus. In severe cases, the vagina becomes impenetrable because the muscles are so contracted. This makes sexual intercourse or inserting anything into the vagina, such as a tampon, difficult or impossible. The cause of vaginismus is usually pyschological—it may stem from a traumatic sexual experience, the anticipation of pain during intercourse, or simply not wanting intercourse.

Conventional treatment may consist of counseling to try to solve a possible psychological cause. Natural remedies that may help include mental and physical relaxation techniques, and sex therapy.

Relaxation
Since the cause of this problem is usually emotional, you may find that anything that promotes mental and physical relaxation will also help you ease your anxieties about vaginal penetration. Regular meditation, progressive relaxation, yoga, or deep-breathing exercises may relax you.

Massage
If you suffer from mild vaginismus, you may find that a sensual massage from your partner before you have intercourse can help you relax so that penetration becomes easier. Use an essential oil such as ylang-ylang or lavender diluted with a base oil such as almond oil.

Sex therapy
When you are relaxed, gently insert the tip of your finger into the vagina and breathe slowly and deeply. Repeat this process in stages over a matter of days until you can insert two or three fingers into the vagina

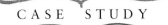

A Woman Who Self-diagnoses

Treating yourself for a gynecological problem without first receiving a medical diagnosis can be dangerous. What seems to be a minor or transient symptom may be a sign of a more serious underlying condition. If you have a symptom such as vaginal discharge that keeps coming back, or if you are feeling under the weather for no apparent reason, see a doctor.

Martha is a 41-year-old single parent whose time is split between her young daughter and her design business, leaving little time for anything else. She is overweight but otherwise generally healthy.

When she developed an irritating vaginal discharge, Martha thought she had a yeast infection. She bought some live-culture yogurt and applied this for a few days. Although the symptoms passed, they reappeared shortly after, coupled with fatigue and lethargy. She treated herself again with yogurt and multivitamin supplements, but this time to no avail.

Lately Martha has realized that she has been losing weight. This is suprising, particularly because she constantly feels hungry and thirsty.

WHAT MARTHA SHOULD DO

Martha has troublesome symptoms, which she attributes to a passing vaginal infection. However, her recurring symptoms are signs that the problem is not one that she should be dealing with herself. She should also be aware that her feelings of fatigue and lethargy may also indicate a more serious medical condition.

Treating herself at home with live-culture yogurt is sensible as a short-term self-help measure, but when it fails to work, it is vital that Martha seek medical help.

Martha should realize that losing weight without changing her diet, eating less, or exercising more means that she should see her doctor immediately.

Action Plan

LIFESTYLE
Concentrate on getting enough rest and relaxation. Stop self-treatment. Make an appointment with a doctor to discuss symptoms as soon as possible.

DIET
Set aside time to eat healthfully and consult a doctor about possible changes in diet.

HEALTH
Take persistent symptoms seriously. Consider the possibility that weight loss, fatigue, and vaginal discharge are connected. Discuss these with a doctor.

DIET
A diet that is high in saturated fat and sugary foods can make you vulnerable, not only to yeast infections but also to more serious illnesses.

HEALTH
When you are busy you may fail to notice that your body is giving you warning signs of illness. This can have serious consequences for your health.

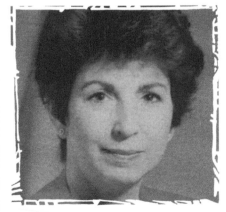

LIFESTYLE
Busy individuals may not allow time to consult a doctor, but self-diagnosis can be dangerous.

HOW THINGS TURNED OUT FOR MARTHA

Eventually Martha visited her family doctor. She was shocked when urine and blood tests revealed mild diabetes mellitus. Her doctor recommended a special diet and referred her to a diabetic clinic. The new diet reduced her blood sugar levels and eased feelings of hunger and thirst.

She used antifungal vaginal suppositories to treat her yeast infection and is now symptom-free. Her experience shows that persistent symptoms require expert help.

AVOIDING PELVIC INFLAMMATORY DISEASE

PID is serious—untreated, it can lead to infertility. The following steps will help you avoid PID.

▶ *After a bowel movement always wipe from front to back to prevent bacteria from being transferred from the anus to the vagina.*

▶ *If you use an IUD, speak to your doctor about the likelihood of infection.*

▶ *If you have multiple sexual partners, you are more likely to contract a sexually transmitted disease. Be sure that your partner(s) wears a condom for protection. Do this even if you are already using another form of birth control.*

comfortably. If vaginal spasms occur, go back to the first stage of the exercise—above all take things slowly and make sure you are relaxed. It may help if you lubricate your fingers with a water-soluble lubricating jelly.

Visualization of lovemaking situations also may help. Combining erotic thoughts and fantasies with the image of being penetrated may promote an association between arousal and penetration. To master these techniques, consult a sex therapist.

PELVIC INFLAMMATORY DISEASE (PID)

PID occurs when the female reproductive organs become infected, causing pelvic pain, fever, and vaginal discharge. It may be either an acute or chronic condition in which the pain is worse following menstruation or during sexual intercourse. Other symptoms may include frequent and painful urination; vaginal bleeding during or after sex, or between periods; swollen abdomen; and general malaise. Seek medical advice immediately if you have any of these symptoms. The cause of PID is not always clearly identifiable, but it may be the result of chlamydia (a microorganism infection of the genital tract), or another sexually transmitted disease, or a complication of childbirth or a miscarriage.

PID is a serious illness that needs correct medical treatment. A doctor will prescribe bed rest, antibiotics, and painkillers. Natural remedies include hydrotherapy to ease immediate symptoms, and acupuncture and naturopathy to treat chronic forms of the disease.

Hydrotherapy

A hot bath or a hot water bottle placed on the abdomen can relieve the pain of PID. The heat will also increase the blood flow to the area and help the body eliminate toxins. You must be

HEAT TREATMENT FOR PID
Once you are sure that your abdominal pains are due to pelvic inflammatory disease you may be able to ease them with a hot water bottle placed on your abdomen.

sure that the pain is not due to another condition in which a direct application of heat may be harmful. A severely inflamed appendix, for example, may rupture if heat is applied to the lower abdomen.

Acupuncture

If you suffer from chronic PID, acupuncture may help. Acupuncturists believe that treatment can direct your body's healing energies to fight the infection.

Naturopathy

Many therapists believe that high doses of vitamin C—at least 1 gram a day—may help to strengthen the immune system.

PROLAPSE OF THE UTERUS

When the uterus is no longer supported by surrounding ligaments and muscles it drops down into the vagina. This condition is called a uterine prolapse and can cause intense discomfort. Pelvic muscles can sometimes weaken as a result of childbirth, the natural aging process, or injury, or it may be an inherited condition.

There are different degrees of prolapse. In mild cases, the cervix begins to descend slightly into the vagina. In very severe cases, however, the cervix and uterus actually protrude out of the vagina. Although there may be few symptoms, a slight dragging sensation in the pelvis, particularly in more severe cases, coupled with backache and difficulty in bowel movements and urination can occur. Conventional treatment to control the problem may be a support in the form of a ring that is inserted into the vagina to help hold up the uterus. In severe cases, surgery, either to repair the prolapse or to remove the uterus, is recommended. By far the best natural treatment is the maintenance of strong pelvic muscles through regular exercise or yoga.

Exercise

Regular pelvic floor exercises, known as Kegels, can strengthen the musculature that supports the uterus and help to prevent or relieve prolapse. To find the muscles that you need to strengthen, stop for a moment when you are in the middle of emptying your bladder—the muscles that you tense in order to stop the flow of urine are the same ones that give support to your pelvic organs, and a similar action can be employed to exercise these muscles.

To practice Kegel exercises, tense the muscles at the entrance of the vagina in three stages as though ascending in an elevator. At each floor hold for up to 10 seconds. Then let the elevator come down again floor by floor, and repeat the sequence half a dozen times several times a day. It may take three months of regular exercise to improve poor muscle tone, although ideally these exercises should be practiced regularly throughout your adult life.

Yoga
Poses that help to tone the pelvic muscles are helpful in the prevention and relief of uterine prolapse. These can be done in conjunction with movements such as head and shoulder stands that invert gravity and take the strain away from the supporting muscles around the pelvic area.

The cat pose is good for abdominal toning. Kneel on the floor with your hands in line with your knees, and your arms and legs at right angles to your body. Take three slow breaths—expanding the abdomen as you inhale and letting it relax as you exhale. On the fourth inhale, slowly hollow your back, stretch back your neck, and look up at the ceiling. On the next inhale, round your back and drop your head between your arms. Hollow the abdomen and tighten the muscles of the anus. Hold for three seconds at the fullest extension, release on the exhale, and return to the original position. Repeat this exercise six times.

It is important that you never force any part of your body into uncomfortable positions. Suppleness must be built up gradually by gently taking your muscles to their comfortable limit. Whatever your limit, hold the posture for three seconds at its fullest extension, then release and breathe out.

BREAST PAIN
Swollen, tender, sore, or painful breasts are very common and normal symptoms during the week or so before menstruation. This cyclic breast pain is experienced by at least 30 percent of women between the ages of 25 and 50. Breast pain is also common during pregnancy and breast-feeding. Consult your doctor, however, if symptoms occur at other times or are associated with fever and inflammation.

Conventional treatment varies depending on the cause, but for premenstrual breast pain, diuretic drugs, which reduce water retention, contraceptive pills, or danazol may be recommended. Breast infections are

PELVIC FLOOR MUSCLES
The ligaments and muscles of the pelvic floor maintain support for the uterus, vagina, urethra, bladder, and rectum.

The levator ani
are the main pelvic floor muscles.

VAGINAL SUPPORT
The pelvic floor muscles can become weakened and slack due to childbirth or as part of the aging process.

treated with antibiotics such as penicillin. Naturopathy, herbalism, aromatherapy, and acupressure may be helpful in alleviating breast tenderness.

Naturopathy
You should reduce your salt intake, because sodium encourages the body to retain fluid, which will exacerbate premenstrual breast tenderness and discomfort.

It may also be a good idea to cut down on the amount of saturated fat you eat because this may increase the effects of female hormones on the breasts. Examples of foods high in saturated fats are butter, lard, beef, hard cheeses, and whole milk.

Herbalism
Parsley has diuretic properties, making it useful for premenstrual breast soreness; simply chew the raw fresh herb. Alternatively, combine parsley leaves with equal parts of buchu, black haw, and cramp bark. Infuse and drink a cup three times a day. (Avoid buchu and excessive amounts of parsley during pregnancy.) A parsley poultice can also be applied directly to the breasts to relieve soreness. If parsley if unavailable, you can substitute cabbage leaves, which have similar properties. Evening primrose oil capsules may also reduce premenstrual breast pain (see page 122).

Aromatherapy
Add eight drops of geranium oil to a base oil, such as sunflower or almond, and use to massage the breasts. Geranium essential oil has analgesic, tonic, and diuretic properties that can help to gently relieve pain. It can also be used in a bath or a compress to treat painful breasts.

Acupressure
Pressure applied to point Liv 3 may help to ease tender, painful breasts. Apply pressure to both of the feet.

Acupressure for breast pain

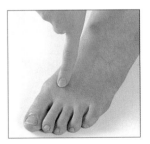

PRESSURE POINT LIV 3
This is found on the foot two finger widths toward the ankle from the junction of the big and second toes.

Self-examination

All women should check their breasts once every month for breast disease. Discovering a lump or other abnormal breast change can result in the early diagnosis and successful treatment of breast cancer.

To examine your breasts properly, you need to be familiar with the way they normally look and feel. As you become used to examining your breasts you will be able to notice any changes quickly and easily. If you do discover anything unusual, see your doctor immediately. Breasts may feel lumpy and tender a week or two before your period, so self-examination should be done the week after menstruation.

1 *Stand in front of a mirror with your arms by your sides. Observe the shape, size, and contour of your breasts. Look for anything unusual, such as an increase in size of one breast or an inverted nipple. Then raise your arms above your head to stretch the skin of the breasts. Look in the mirror for any dimpling. Turn from side to side so that you can see your breasts from all angles.*

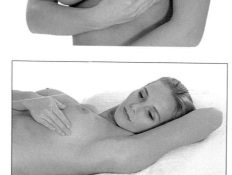

2 *Look down at your breasts and check for any unusual coloring or change in shape around your nipples. Gently squeeze your nipples between your thumb and forefinger. Check that there is no discharge or cracking of the skin, and that your nipple returns easily to its normal shape after you have squeezed it.*

If you notice any discharge when you gently squeeze your nipples, see your doctor immediately.

WHAT TO LOOK FOR

If you notice any of the following changes, you should see your doctor who will thoroughly examine your breasts and may suggest mammography or other tests. This will ensure that any serious problems can be diagnosed and treated as early as possible.

► *An increase in the size of one or both breasts.*

► *A change in the shape of one or both breasts.*

► *Puckering, dimpling, or any change in texture or contour.*

► *A lump or swelling in the breast, armpit, or collarbone.*

► *A newly inverted nipple.*

► *A discharge from the nipples.*

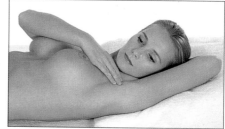

3 *Lie on your back with your head and shoulders supported by a pillow and your left arm by your side. Hold the fingers of your right hand flat and move them in a circular direction around the left breast, pressing down gently. Repeat with your right breast. Now examine your left breast with your left hand behind your head and your right breast with your right hand behind your head.*

4 *For the last step of your self-examination, put your left hand behind your head and, using the fingers of your right hand, gently feel along your collarbone and in your armpits for lumps or swellings. Repeat with your right hand behind your head and use your left hand to examine your collarbone and armpits.*

Pregnancy and Childbirth

Modern maternity care has greatly improved the health and well-being of mothers and babies, but natural remedies are still useful for easing symptoms from morning sickness to baby blues.

The physical and hormonal changes that occur when a woman becomes pregnant can be very disconcerting. Problem-free pregnancies, however, are not unusual and many common complaints can be easily managed.

MORNING SICKNESS

Nausea or vomiting in the first three months of pregnancy is extremely common, but contrary to its name morning sickness may occur at any time of the day, and it can last throughout a pregnancy. Thought to be due to massive changes in hormone levels, morning sickness may vary from mild and intermittent nausea to persistent vomiting. Although unpleasant and uncomfortable, it is unlikely to cause damage to the baby and should certainly not be viewed as a sign of an unhealthy pregnancy.

Conventional medicine has little to offer for fear of affecting the baby, but if severe morning sickness causes dehydration, an intravenous infusion is necessary to replace lost fluids. Of the natural remedies, massaging acupressure points and taking specific herbs and Chinese remedies may relieve symptoms and reduce vomiting.

Acupressure
Apply pressure to point P 6. Use vibrating finger pressure for 20 seconds, then relax.

Herbalism
An infusion of one part black horehound and one part chamomile taken three times every day (or as required) may help relieve morning sickness.

Many people find that ginger taken in tea or capsule form eases nausea. Others find that even ginger ale or gingerroot, an ingredient found in many stir-fried dishes, can relieve a queasy stomach.

Chinese medicine
Your herbalist can make up a personalized prescription for you, or your acupuncturist may be able to reduce the nausea considerably with weekly treatment for the duration of the sickness.

MISCARRIAGE

Most women who miscarry do so in the first 10 weeks of pregnancy, although it can happen as late as 28 weeks. It is estimated that at least half of miscarriages occur because the fetus has become unviable. Other causes may include hormonal imbalances, structural problems in the uterus or cervix, environmental toxins, infection, and emotional or physical trauma.

A miscarriage is usually heralded by cramps or bleeding. In the very early stages of pregnancy it may seem little more than a heavy period and many women may have been unaware that they were pregnant and miscarried. A miscarriage later in a pregnancy is likely to involve a more apparent expulsion of the fetus.

Any bleeding during pregnancy should be treated by a doctor, who will usually advise bed rest. After a miscarriage a procedure called dilatation and curettage (D&C) may be performed to clear the uterus of any remaining placental and fetal material. Homeopathy, herbalism, and Bach flower remedies are said to aid recovery by strengthening the uterus and relieving pain.

Homeopathy
Bellis perennis For uterine healing after having a miscarriage.

Herbalism
If you have suffered previous miscarriages, an herbalist may recommend a "uterine tonic" to try to prevent another miscarriage.

Acupressure for morning sickness

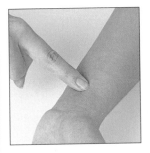

PRESSURE POINT P 6
This point is located in the middle of the inside of the forearm, two to three finger widths up from the wrist crease. The point sits between two tendons that can be found by clenching the fist slightly.

Dietary Remedies

Morning sickness can make the first trimester of a pregnancy uncomfortable. Often a woman's appetite for certain foods changes dramatically. Coffee, alcoholic drinks, and foods with strong flavors and smells may be particularly nauseating.

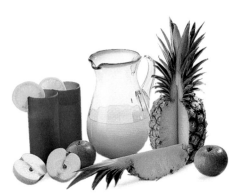

FRESH FRUIT JUICES
A glass of fresh apple or pineapple juice can be a quick remedy for nausea. Keep a glass or jug of juice next to your bed during the night.

The best advice for pregnant women suffering from morning sickness is to follow their instincts about food, but the following dietary advice may help to ease nausea and vomiting.

FOODS TO EAT OR AVOID

Coffee, tea, cola, and chocolate all contain caffeine and are likely to make nausea worse. Sugary foods may be tempting, but can frequently contribute to nausea. Fatty foods may also upset your stomach.

Enlist your family's cooperation in eliminating any foods you find particularly nauseating and try to choose quick-cooking or cold foods that do not have lingering smells or strong tastes, or require a great deal of preparation. Many women find that drinking a glass of apple or pineapple juice helps quell nausea.

Getting out of bed suddenly can bring on nausea, so, if possible, ask someone to bring you a drink and a dry biscuit to eat before you get up in the morning.

Eat small, low-fat meals regularly and frequently, and if you discover a food that is less upsetting than anything else, eat more of it.

If it is hard to keep solid food down, try homemade vegetable or fruit juices, milk drinks, soy milk shakes, and chamomile tea. It is very important that you do not become dehydrated or deficient in essential vitamins and minerals.

NAUSEA RELIEF
A cup of warm ginger tea can help relieve nausea.

GINGER TO EASE NAUSEA

Ginger is a safe and effective remedy for morning sickness and there are various ways of taking it. Many women prefer to drink ginger tea—simply add a teaspoon of grated gingerroot per cup of boiling water.

The tea should steep for about 10 minutes and then may be strained. It is best to drink it while it is still warm. Ginger in any form, even capsules, may be taken as often as necessary to prevent nausea.

Fresh gingerroot should be used.

FRESH GINGER
Finely grate 1 teaspoon of ginger into a glass or a cup.

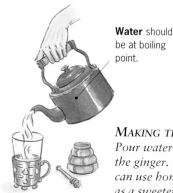

Water should be at boiling point.

MAKING TEA
Pour water over the ginger. You can use honey as a sweetener.

This may consist of an infusion of two parts false unicorn root and one part cramp bark. You should consult an herbalist about appropriate herbal medicines rather than treating yourself at home.

Bach flower remedies

To treat the shock of a threatened miscarriage, a few drops of rescue remedy straight on the tongue may help relax you. Many threats of miscarriage are simply that, and often rest and relaxation will solve the problem. Rock rose, taken four times daily, may help ease feelings of fear or panic.

LABOR PAINS

The degree of pain experienced during childbirth varies from one woman to another. Personal and cultural attitudes toward childbirth, knowledge of its stages, and one's expectations have been found to be very influential. The pain experienced at the end of pregnancy begins with uterine contractions that open the cervix in preparation for childbirth. These are followed by the contractions that move the baby down and out of the birth canal and expel the placenta.

Doctors now encourage natural childbirth or techniques that use breathing patterns to control pain. A variety of painkilling drugs may also be used in conjunction with natural childbirth, if necessary.

One type of pain relief is an epidural, which is an anesthetic given in the lower spine to numb the entire pelvic area. This proves satisfactory for some women, but there is evidence that epidurals may cause low blood pressure in the mother and lack of responsiveness in the newborn baby. These effects, however, will not last for any length of time.

The natural therapies that can be used instead of or in conjunction with orthodox pain relief during labor include aromatherapy, massage, homeopathy, acupressure, specific breathing techniques, acupuncture, and transcutaneous electrical nerve stimulation (TENS).

Aromatherapy

A gentle massage of the sacrum, the large triangular bone at the base of the spine, by your partner or birth assistant can soothe labor pains. Four to six drops of clary sage or lavender essential oil should be combined with a carrier oil (see page 21) and applied in light strokes in a clockwise direction. The entire spine can also be massaged from the bottom to the top in even rhythmic strokes, working from the spine outward.

Massage

Talcum powder can be used instead of oil to massage the buttocks and back. Apply slow, firm strokes from the center of the lower back moving out to the sides and gradually moving up the spine.

Very light circular pressure, or simply leaning with gentle pressure on the lower spine, can give relief during contractions. Many women find that gentle neck stroking brings relief throughout childbirth.

Homeopathy

Nux vomica For sudden spasms of pain with impatience and anger.
Coffea For hypersensitivity to touch, light, and noise.
Pulsatilla For being hot and weepy and needing reassurance.
Aconite For fear and panic.

Acupressure

To encourage contractions and relieve pain, apply pressure to Sp 6 (see page 128), which can be found just off the edge of the shinbone, three finger widths above the ankle. This is likely to be tender, so it is best to use only gentle pressure. If you feel depressed or irritable, massage Liv 3 (see page 131), two finger widths toward the ankle from the junction of the big and second toes. To encourage the baby to be born, massage LI 4 (see page 68), which is found in the webbing between the forefinger and thumb. To reduce pain stimulate point Bl 60.

Breathing techniques

During the early stages of labor, concentrate on slow deep breathing. Breathe out through your mouth at the beginning of the contraction and breathe in through your nose. As the contractions become more intense, make your breathing light and shallow. Breathe in and out quickly through your mouth at the height of the pain, but be careful not to hyperventilate. Classes that teach various breathing techniques in preparation for labor are widely offered by nurses, midwives, hospitals, and childbirth education organizations.

Acupuncture and TENS

Although acupressure can help during labor, a more dramatic result may be obtained with acupuncture and, to a lesser degree, with transcutaneous electrical nerve stimulation (TENS—see page 26). Treatment may be specially tailored to speed or

Acupressure for labor pains

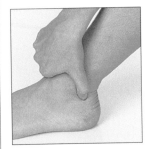

PRESSURE POINT BL 60 This is located between the outer ankle bone and the Achilles tendon.

Natural birthing positions

Studies have found that a prone position can increase the length of labor and the risk of distress to the baby, while decreasing the strength and efficiency of contractions.

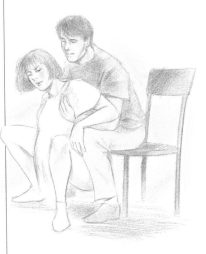

UPRIGHT CHILDBIRTH Squatting, standing, kneeling, or using a birthing chair are all suitable alternatives to lying down.

PREVENTING NIPPLE PROBLEMS

The following suggestions may help to prevent sore nipples while breast-feeding.

▶ *Make sure that the baby latches on properly to the nipple so that the nipple does not move around in the baby's mouth.*

▶ *Let the nipple dry naturally with a little milk on it after the baby has finished nursing.*

▶ *Wash your nipples with baby lotion rather than soap, and apply cocoa butter to them.*

BREAST-FEEDING
Your nipples may become tender when you first start to breast-feed, but this will ease over time.

slow contractions, reduce pain, ease delivery, expel the placenta, and even encourage lactation. Many acupuncturists will attend a delivery upon request; you may want to choose one who is specially trained in obstetrical acupuncture.

BREAST-FEEDING PROBLEMS

Most women will generally experience problem-free breast-feeding, but some may produce too much or too little milk. With overproduction, breasts become engorged. This can be relieved by expressing your milk by hand and storing or discarding it.

Not producing enough milk is less easy to recognize and not so easily remedied. As a general rule, if your baby wets fewer than six diapers a day, he or she is not getting enough milk. Monitor the baby very carefully because dehydration can quickly become a dangerous problem.

Herbalism and naturopathy may help if you are producing an inadequate supply of milk; homeopathy may help both problems.
Herbalism
Dandelion root may increase milk production: use 1 teaspoon per cup of water, boil for 10 minutes, and drink three times a day.
Naturopathy
Eat plenty of whole-grain cereals; fruits, especially those high in vitamin C such as strawberries; vegetables; and low-fat protein such as chicken. Also drink plenty of fluids.
Homeopathy
Pulsatilla For breasts that are swollen as a result of weaning very quickly.
Aconite For loss of milk due to shock.
Calcarea carbonica For excess milk production accompanied by feeling cold and cold sweats (take hourly for six doses).
Agnus castus For milk loss.

PAINFUL BREASTS

Sore or painful nipples are common among mothers who have just started breast-feeding, although it is likely to become less of a problem as feeding proceeds and your nipples are not as tender. Mastitis is an inflammation of the breast tissue that causes pain, tenderness, and swelling, along with fever and chills. Mastitis may be caused by bacteria that enter the breast through a crack in the nipple. It must be treated by a doctor who will prescribe antibiotics.

The infection usually clears up in 48 hours, but may lead to an abscess, a localized infection that must be surgically drained. Homeopathy or hydrotherapy may relieve the discomfort of painful breasts.
Homeopathy
Chamomilla For inflamed nipples that are painful to touch.
Sulfur For cracked nipples accompanied by smarting, burning pain.
Bryonia For hot, hard, painful breasts.
Hydrotherapy
Warm compresses may help relieve discomfort due to mastitis.

POSTPARTUM DEPRESSION

After childbirth it is common for women to experience an emotional low, commonly known as the baby blues. This is caused by a sudden change in hormone levels shortly after giving birth, often coupled with fatigue and perhaps feelings of inadequacy for the responsibility of a newborn. Weepiness, moodiness, and anxiety may last a week or two. Doctors do not generally treat the condition unless it is prolonged and characterized by lack of interest in life or the child, or, in more severe cases, thoughts of suicide.

Conventional treatment usually consists of antidepressant drugs, unless the mother is nursing, and counseling or psychotherapy. Postpartum depression may also respond to the natural remedies given below.
Herbalism
St. John's wort, taken as a supplement, may help to alleviate depression.
Aromatherapy
To elevate mood, therapists advocate adding a few drops of clary sage, geranium, or ylang-ylang to bathwater. A massage with a base oil containing a few drops of rosemary, lavender, or chamomile oil can also help.
Naturopathy
A deficiency of zinc, magnesium, and the B vitamins can contribute to postpartum depression; consult a doctor or naturopath about taking them as dietary supplements.
Bach flower remedies
Try a combination of mimulus for fear, and rock rose, walnut, and star-of-Bethlehem for panic. Make a remedy and take a couple of drops on the tongue as required.
Chinese medicine
A combination of acupuncture, moxibustion (see page 28), and Chinese herbs may help to restore balance in the body. Consult a doctor of Chinese medicine.

MENOPAUSE

The physical symptoms of menopause are caused by hormonal fluctuations and vary in severity from woman to woman. Many natural remedies are available to ease discomfort.

Menopause is the cessation of menstruation. However, prior to this event is a period of months or years during which the female hormones, estrogen and progesterone, are produced in fluctuating amounts. These fluctuations can cause troublesome symptoms.

HOT FLASHES

The most common symptom of menopause is the hot flash. Aberrations in the autonomic nervous system, which regulates blood vessels, cause these vessels to dilate and fill with blood. This leads to a rush of heat to the head and neck, sometimes the whole body, which lasts between three and five minutes and may be accompanied by sweating and reddened skin. Hot flashes may occur occasionally or up to several times an hour. In severe cases, women suffer from frequent hot flashes for several years. As the body adjusts to lower estrogen levels, flashes usually subside.

Conventional medical treatment for hot flashes centers around hormone replacement therapy (HRT), in which natural or synthetic forms of estrogen and progesterone are used to restore the female hormones to their premenopausal levels. HRT is usually prescribed by doctors in pill form, but skin patches, implants, creams, and injections are also available. Natural alternatives or complements to HRT include homeopathy, acupressure, and naturopathy.

Homeopathy
Lachesis For hot flashes that affect the head and face.
Sepia For hot flashes accompanied by anxiety attacks.
Pulsatilla For hot flashes together with sweating on the face.
Belladonna For a sweaty face.

Acupressure
As a hot flash begins, try massaging Liv 2 (see page 124). This is the point at the junc-ture of the big toe and the second toe. This may cool you down by drawing heat away from the top of the body.

To prevent hot flashes, try massaging either Liv 3 (see page 131), which is two finger widths up from the juncture between the big and second toe, or Sp 6 (see page 128), which is three finger widths up from the ankle bone, just off the edge of the shinbone. Acupuncture may also be useful for relieving hot flashes.

Naturopathy
Vitamin E is thought to help relieve some menopausal symptoms, especially hot flashes and night sweats (consult a doctor before taking vitamin E if you have diabetes, high blood pressure, or heart disease). Natural sources include leafy greens, vegetable oils, nuts, and wheat germ. Very hot drinks and spicy foods can trigger hot flashes, so cut down on them or avoid them completely.

NIGHT SWEATS

Hormonal changes also cause some menopausal women to have night sweats. These are a variation of hot flashes, characterized by spontaneous sweating that may be profuse and disrupt sleep. Feeling chilled after suffering a night sweat is common, and severe ones may cause insomnia. It is important that night sweats are correctly diagnosed because they can be symptomatic of other, more serious, diseases. If you have any doubts about them, see your doctor.

The frequency of night sweats varies for individuals, from isolated occasions to sev-

EASING NIGHT SWEATS
Keep a bowl of water and a sponge or washcloth near your bed. Applying lavender water to the face is cooling. An electric fan may help to cool your room.

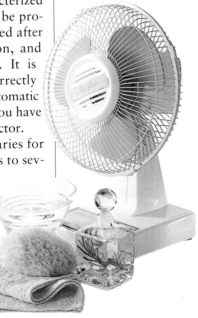

HELP FOR HOT FLASHES

Many women suffer from hot flashes and night sweats. There are several ways to reduce their frequency and severity.

▶ *Try to plan ahead so that you do not have to rush around.*

▶ *Wear clothes made of natural fibers.*

▶ *Wear clothes that can be unbuttoned or layers that you can take off. Avoid tight or high-necked clothing.*

▶ *Do not overheat your rooms and, if possible, keep a window open.*

▶ *During a hot flash, sit down somewhere quiet and practice visualization (see page 30).*

Relieving Menopausal Complaints with

Herbal Remedies

Hot flashes, night sweats, insomnia, and fatigue can cause discomfort for several years. Treating these symptoms with a homemade herbal preparation can help you manage your menopause and give you a sense of control.

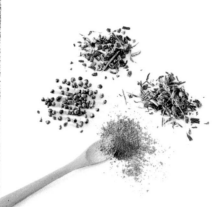

HERBS FOR MENOPAUSE
Goldenseal, St. John's wort, chaste tree, and black cohosh are particularly recommended to help ease the various symptoms brought about by menopause.

Chaste tree (also known as *Vitex agnus-castus*) is good for most menopausal symptoms. Infuse 1 teaspoon of the dried berries, either store-bought or gathered (as with all the herbs), in a cup of boiling water for 15 minutes. Drink three times a day.

Black cohosh has a normalizing effect on hormone production and eases aching joints. Unearth the roots in fall and dry them. Add a cup of water to 1 teaspoon of the root, simmer for 15 minutes, then drink.

Goldenseal may be helpful for heavy menopausal periods (should not be used if you may be pregnant).

The roots of three-year-old plants should be dried, prepared, and taken in the same way as black cohosh.

Oats may be helpful for general debility, exhaustion, and depression and can be eaten as oatmeal, or you can pick the stems, leaves, and grains when ripe and prepare them in the same way as black cohosh.

St. John's wort may help alleviate irritability and anxiety (substitute motherwort if you have high blood pressure or heart palpitations). Gather the flowers, stems, and leaves and dry them. Prepare in the same way as chaste tree.

CALENDULA OINTMENT RECIPE

It is common for menopausal women to suffer dryness and inflammation of the vagina and vulva. This may be remedied with an ointment made from calendula flowers (marigold).

Calendula is believed to have certain astringent and antiseptic properties that may help to relieve irritation or infection, while the oils may help to remoisturize dry, itchy skin.

HEAT THE INGREDIENTS
Melt 2 ounces of lanolin and 2 fluid ounces (¼ cup) of wheat germ oil. Add a handful of fresh or dried calendula flowers; simmer for about two hours.

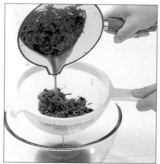

STRAIN THE MIXTURE
Remove the pan from the heat and strain through muslin or a sieve, retaining the liquid.

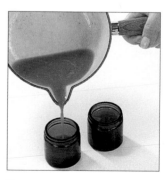

LEAVE TO SET
Stir in two capsules of vitamin E, pour into sterilized containers, and leave to set. Use as required.

eral times a night. Hormone replacement therapy will relieve night sweats, but hydrotherapy is a natural alternative that will quickly cool your body temperature.

Hydrotherapy

Tepid sponging can help to cool your face and chest when you wake up feeling feverish. Simply soak a sponge or washcloth in tepid or cool water—not cold water because this causes the small blood vessels beneath the skin to constrict, a mechanism that works to preserve body heat.

If you suffer from frequent night sweats, a naturopath may recommend a hydrotherapy treatment in which alternating hot and cold jets of water are directed up and down the spine. This stimulates the circulation, cooling the blood nearest the surface of the skin, and leaves you with a pleasant, invigorating, tingling sensation.

VAGINAL DRYNESS

When estrogen levels decline at menopause, the tissues of the vagina and vulva begin to dry out and become thin and less elastic. Known as genital atrophy, this can cause discomfort and itchiness, as well as making sexual intercourse uncomfortable and vaginal infections and irritations more likely.

Doctors generally prescribe hormone replacement therapy for severe dryness of the vagina, but often a local application of estrogen, in cream or suppository form, is sufficient. Homeopathic remedies, naturopathy, and Chinese medicine—both herbs and acupuncture—may also aid in combating vaginal dryness.

Homeopathy

Sepia For a dry vagina, accompanied by hot flashes and thinning hair, especially if there is a risk of uterine prolapse.
Sulfur For a red, dry, itchy vagina and burning sensations.
Pulsatilla For vaginal dryness and discharge, particularly if accompanied by mood swings and tearfulness.

Naturopathy

Vitamin E is thought to promote chemical activities similar to those activated by estrogen, which makes it useful during menopause. It can be taken as a supplement, but consult your doctor before taking it if you have heart disease or hypertension. Foods that contain vitamin E, like whole-grain cereals and nuts, should be included in your daily diet.

Chinese medicine

A Chinese doctor may prescribe herbs and a course of acupuncture to alleviate vaginal dryness. Dang Gui (Chinese angelica) and Bai Shao Yao (white peony root) are commonly prescribed as herbal remedies.

SKIN AND HAIR CHANGES

During the years after menopause the collagen and elastin fibers that give skin its suppleness and strength gradually disintegrate, and the skin becomes thinner and more prone to wrinkling. The hair may also begin to thin and the nails become dry and brittle.

One of the best ways to take care of skin is to stay out of direct sunlight, and use a sunscreen rated SPF 15 or higher whenever you spend more than a few minutes in the sun. Prolonged exposure to the sun's ultraviolet rays increases the risk of developing skin cancer and accelerates wrinkling.

Dry, itchy skin can also be a problem. As you age, the rate of skin cell replacement slows, and dry, dead cells tend to stay on the surface longer, often causing itchiness. Using moisturizing lotions, avoiding hot

AVOIDING VAGINAL DRYNESS

When the vagina lacks lubrication it becomes prone to itchiness and infection. There are measures you can take to keep your vagina from becoming too dry.

▶ *Clean the genital area with plain water, gentle unperfumed soap, or baby oil. Rinse well after washing.*

▶ *Do not use perfumed douches.*

▶ *Regular sexual activity can help to keep the vagina naturally lubricated.*

▶ *Use a lubricating jelly or a vaginal moisturizer if intercourse is uncomfortable or painful.*

HEALTHY SKIN, HAIR, AND NAILS

Moisturizing dry skin twice daily with a cream that contains alpha hydroxy, or fruit, acids (AHAs) will help to diminish fine lines and wrinkles. To keep your nails and hands in good condition, use a cream that contains almond oil. Both skin and hair respond well to a diet that is free from caffeine and alcohol and high in whole grains and fresh fruits and vegetables.

VITAMIN SUPPLEMENTS, especially vitamins A, C, and E (the antioxidants), may help to offset the damage to skin from sun, cigarette smoking, and the normal aging process.

A moisturizer will hydrate skin.

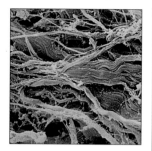

CONNECTIVE FIBERS
Bundles of healthy collagen and elastin fibers support the body's tissues and organs. After menopause these connective fibers lose their strength and suppleness, resulting in wrinkled skin.

water and strong soap, and limiting exposure to cold, dry air and wind can help alleviate discomfort. The natural remedies below may also be useful.

Hydrotherapy
Alternating hot and cold water can nourish the skin by improving circulation. After a hot shower, a brief cold shower will invigorate skin, close the pores, and encourage the elimination of toxins.

Herbalism
Herbs with antioxidant properties, such as horse chestnut and witch hazel, are good for fighting wrinkles. So, too, is Aloe vera gel, which restores damaged skin and softens it. Pureed cucumber and mashed avocado make excellent moisturizers for the face. And olive oil, though not an herb, has for centuries been used to keep skin soft and moist.

OSTEOPOROSIS
Osteoporosis, a disease in which bones lose calcium and other minerals, is a major concern after menopause. Among people with advanced cases, wrist and hip fractures are common. Hormone replacement therapy is the standard treatment, but diet and exercise also play important roles (see page 108).

REDUCED SEXUAL PLEASURE
Diminished libido in menopausal women may be due to emotional symptoms, such as anxiety and depression, or physical symptoms, such as night sweats and insomnia, but often it is caused by vaginal dryness that makes sexual intercourse painful.

Doctors usually prescribe hormone replacement therapy or an estrogen cream to increase vaginal lubrication. If you do not wish to use estrogen, regular sensual massage from your partner may improve lubrication and increase sexual pleasure by giving your body time to respond naturally. A water-based lubricating jelly or long-lasting moisturizer applied to the vagina also can be helpful.

Sensual massage
You and your partner can take advantage of the slower sexual response that both men and women experience as they age by making the buildup to lovemaking longer and more sensual. Use your imagination to think of techniques that will enhance and lengthen foreplay. Sensual massage and sensate focus (see page 145) are ideal ways of doing this. There is no right or wrong way to practice sensual massage. Try starting with your partner's feet, stroking, rubbing, caressing, and kissing. Responding to your partner's likes, move up the legs and thighs. The abdomen can be massaged gently in a clockwise circle, and then the chest, shoulders, and arms. Most people enjoy receiving a back massage, especially with an essential oil diluted in a carrier oil—ylang-ylang, jasmine, or neroli are all thought to have aphrodisiac properties.

Regular sexual activity can increase blood flow to the pelvic tissues, tone pelvic muscles, and increase vaginal secretions.

STRESS INCONTINENCE
Sometimes the muscles and tissues supporting the bladder or urethra become thin and stretched and the urethra or bladder drops down and bulges into the vaginal wall. The result may be frequent urinary infections or a mild type of incontinence known as stress incontinence. The main symptom is a small leakage of urine when stress—for example, strenuous exercise, laughing, coughing, or sneezing—is placed on the bladder.

Conventional treatment includes HRT, which thickens the tissues of the vagina, and urinary tract surgery to repair a prolapsed bladder or urethra. Mild stress incontinence can often be cured with Kegel exercises.

Exercise
To strengthen the muscles used for controlling the bladder, practice the Kegel exercises on page 130. For them to be really effective you should do 20 to 30 repetitions three or four times a day for at least three months and should continue them for the rest of your life.

Kegel exercises help tone the pubococcygeal muscles, and since these muscles are also associated with the vagina, strengthening the muscles in this area may improve your sexual enjoyment as well.

MANAGING STRESS INCONTINENCE

Empty your bladder every two hours, even if you do not need to. If you feel the need to urinate within two hours, stay still, relax, and practice Kegel exercises. After the urge has gone, go to the toilet. Avoid drinking large amounts of fluid if you are not going to be near a toilet.

CHAPTER 10

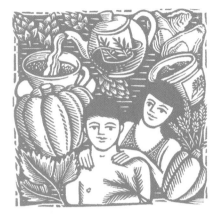

MEN'S HEALTH

Although men do not experience the same range of problems affecting the urogenital tract as women, they are vulnerable to psychosexual problems such as premature ejaculation and impotence. The prostate gland is also susceptible to inflammation and infection and, particularly in old age, enlargement. Therapies that can be used to treat these problems include herbalism, naturopathy, and exercise.

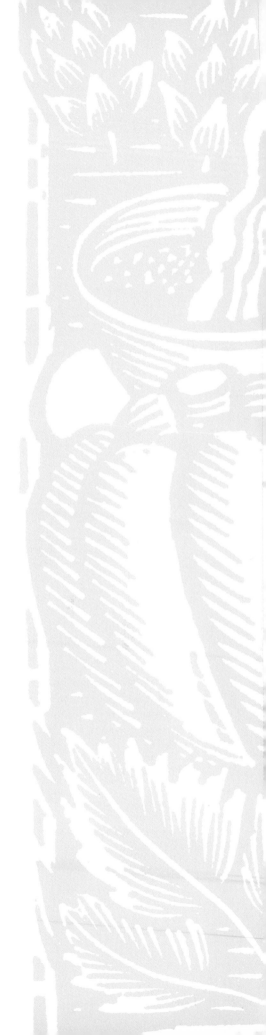

SEXUAL PROBLEMS

Premature ejaculation, a reduced sex drive, and impotence affect sexual performance. Fortunately, there are both natural and conventional treatments available.

Sexual difficulties for men are often age related. Premature ejaculation, for example, may be a problem for young men who are sexually inexperienced, whereas problems with sexual drive tend to affect older men, whether due to physical or emotional reasons. Low sex drive is common to both men and women.

PREMATURE EJACULATION

When a man persistently ejaculates before, upon, or shortly after penetration, he is said to be ejaculating prematurely. Two common causes are anxiety about sex and inexperience in controlling ejaculation.

If premature ejaculation is associated with psychological problems, deep-rooted fears, anxieties, or inhibitions about sex, then pyschosexual counseling may be required. Herbalism, homeopathy, and sex therapy may also offer treatments to help prevent and delay premature ejaculation.

Herbalism

For premature ejaculation caused by anxiety, some herbalists recommend a standard infusion of hops three times a day. Do not take hops if you suffer from depression, because they act as a mild depressant.

Homeopathy

Lycopodium For premature ejaculation brought on by worry or fear of failure.
Nux vomica For premature ejaculation due to impatience and stress.

Sex therapy

The stop and start technique, taught by sex therapists, involves the manual stimulation of the penis by a partner. When you feel you are approaching orgasm, tell your partner to stop stimulating you. After 30 to 60 seconds resume stimulation, but stop again before orgasm. Repeat this three times before allowing ejaculation. If you perform this exercise with your partner you should gradually develop better control.

REDUCED SEX DRIVE

Libido or sexual desire is a difficult thing to measure, but if you feel less interested in sex than you used to be, or find it difficult to become or remain aroused, then you may be suffering from reduced sex drive.

Some physical causes of low sex drive include hormone imbalance, chronic disease, certain medications, alcohol, tobacco, or recent surgery. If you have problems in your relationship, are suffering from depression, or are preoccupied with work, the condition of your house, or financial problems, then all of these are likely to have an adverse effect on your sex life.

There are few conventional treatments for low sex drive, although your doctor may refer you for sex therapy or counseling.

Several herbal preparations are reputed to be aphrodisiacs. Acupressure, massage, and relaxation may also help increase sex drive.

MALE UROGENITAL TRACT

The urethra is a narrow tube that carries urine from the bladder, and semen from the testicles, out of the body via the penis. The penis consists of cylindrical bodies of erectile tissue, through which the urethra carries the fluids.

THE MALE UROGENITAL TRACT
Sperm—the male sex cells in semen—are manufactured and stored in the testicles. They are then passed through the prostate gland, where secretions are added to them. The semen is ejaculated via the urethra in the penis.

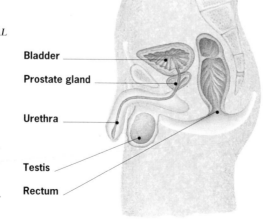

Bladder

Prostate gland

Urethra

Testis

Rectum

HERBS TO RESTORE SEX DRIVE

This recipe is recommended by some herbalists to help both men and women revive sexual desire. You can make a batch of the mixture and store it until you are ready to use it. Don't take this remedy if you suffer from high blood pressure.

▶ *Place 1 to 3 roots of ginseng, 1 ounce damiana, 1 ounce saw palmetto, 2 ounces wild yam, 2 ounces licorice, and 2 ounces St. John's wort in a 1-quart jar.*

▶ *Cover the herbal mixture completely with brandy and seal with an airtight lid.*

▶ *Leave the jar in a warm, dark place for at least six weeks.*

▶ *Strain and save the liquid and the ginseng roots. Discard the rest of the mixture.*

▶ *To each cup of the liquid add half a cup of black cherry concentrate and the ginseng from the original mixture.*

▶ *Store the elixir in the refrigerator and take 1 tablespoon every day.*

▶ *If you find the mixture unpalatable, mix in a little honey to sweeten it.*

Acupressure
Apply pressure to Bl 23 (see page 41). You can find this point on the lower back, between the second and third lumbar vertebrae two finger widths away from the spine at waist level. It may be easier to ask your partner to massage Bl 23 for you, using some scented massage oil.

Massage
Mix together fragranced oils (a suggested combination is one drop each of ylang-ylang, sandalwood, and jasmine essential oils added to a carrier oil such as almond) and use them in sensual massage.

Relaxation
If your difficulties are due to stress or anxiety, relaxation may help. Practise tai chi, yoga, or deep breathing.

IMPOTENCE
Most of the time, impotence—the inability to attain or sustain an erection—is a temporary and common response to stress, fatigue, or drinking excessive amounts of alcohol.

Other possible causes include medical conditions like diabetes mellitus and spinal cord injury, some medications, and certain surgical procedures.

If you are unable to achieve an erection under any circumstances, there may be a physical cause and you should see a doctor.

Conventional help includes the treatment of any underlying medical problem, counseling for emotional difficulties, or, in severe cases, penile implants or injections.

Western and Chinese herbalism claim remedies for impotence. Exercising the pubococcygeal muscles, which run from the pubic bone to the coccyx, and eating a healthy diet may help.

Herbalism
If impotence is due to an organic dysfunction, herbalists may recommend *Ginkgo biloba*, taken in the form of tablets of standardized ginkgo extract, to increase peripheral circulation of blood to the penis.

Yohimbine extract is made from the bark of the Pausinystalia yohimbe tree. It may be effective for impotence that has psychological origins, but side effects have been recorded, so it must be taken under the guidance of a doctor. (Anyone suffering from hypertension should not take yohimbine.)

Chinese herbalism
Traditionally, impotence is thought to be due to deficient Kidney Yin or Yang. A Yin tonic, such as Gou Qi Zi (wolfberry), or a Yang tonic, such as Yin Yang Huo (goat's wort), is given to replenish fluids and energy.

Exercise
A set of exercises, called Kegels, which concentrate on the pubococcygeal muscle, may sustain erections and sexual endurance and benefit the prostate gland. To locate this muscle, start to urinate and then stop in midflow. The muscle you have tensed is the pubococcygeal (PC) muscle.

Exercise this muscle daily. Contract it, hold it clenched, and count slowly to three, and relax. Then clench and relax as fast as you can, and relax. Repeat, starting with 10 to 15 contractions twice a day and working up to 60 to 70 contractions each session.

Naturopathy
Prolactin, a hormone produced by the pituitary gland, inhibits testosterone production. Eating up to 3 ounces (¼ to ½ cup) of sunflower or pumpkin seeds, which contain essential fatty acids and zinc, each day can reduce prolactin levels. Other substances, such as beer, increase prolactin levels and should be avoided. Beer also contains hops which have an estrogenic activity (a female hormone) and may decrease male sex drive.

ALCOHOL AND YOUR SEX DRIVE
Too much alcohol can kill your sexual drive. Beer is particularly damaging because it has a high hops content. Hops have an effect similar to that of estrogen, the female sex hormone, which in men can depress sex drive.

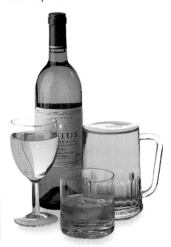

The Sex Therapist

Therapists are professional counselors who treat sexual problems that are psychological rather than physiological in origin. Low sex drive is amenable to treatment with therapies such as sensate focus.

THE THERAPY
A therapist will spend time with you and your partner discussing problem areas in your relationship and sex life. These sessions may then be continued, or may develop into individual counseling sessions where you and your partner are seen separately.

A sex therapist is specially trained to teach couples and individuals how to overcome sexual difficulties by changing their sensual approaches and sexual behavior.

What are the most common problems treated by a sex therapist?
In a study published in the 1970's, most sex therapists reported that the main problems they encountered

were concerned either with male erection or female orgasm. *The Kinsey Institute New Report on Sex* (1990) states that almost half of all patients have problems with sexual desire, or low sex drive, although the majority still claim that physical symptoms are the problem.

What happens at the first session?
Initially the therapist will take a sexual history of the individual or couple. Detailed questions will be asked, including what messages about sex the person learned when young; when the person started to be sexually active; what his or her early sex life was like; if the person masturbates; and what sort of sexual relationships have been experienced.

The individual or couple will also be asked questions about health, current medications, and any recent surgery. In some cases, a client may be asked to have a physical examination by a doctor. This is to eliminate the possibility of an underlying physical problem.

How long does sex therapy take?
Depending on the severity of the problem, treatment can range from a single session to a course of sessions ranging over six months. On average treatment lasts from 12 to 16 biweekly hour-long sessions.

What kind of treatment is used for low sex drive?
Men and women with low sexual desire should first be medically screened before sex therapy is

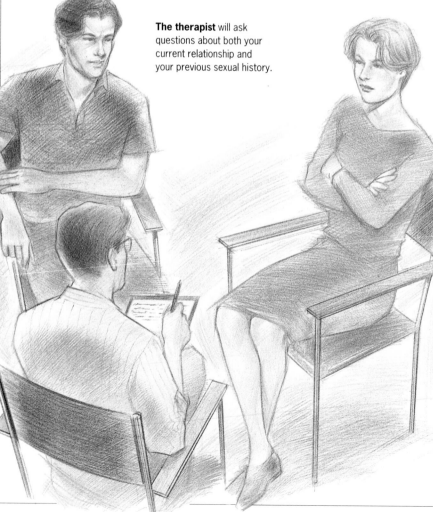

The therapist will ask questions about both your current relationship and your previous sexual history.

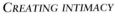

MASSAGE
With sensate focus—a form of massage— learn how to please your partner sexually.

attempted, because if there is any underlying medical cause (see page 142), counseling will not help.

If you consult a sex therapist and there is no physical cause for the problem, your treatment may include masturbation techniques and sexual fantasy, or you may be invited to attend a therapy group. Couples who

consult a sex therapist may be asked to practice a therapy known as sensate focus at home between counseling sessions.

What is sensate focus?
A type of massage, sensate focus helps men and women literally get in touch with each other and discover pleasurable sensations involved in intimate physical contact.

Couples may be asked to spend at least two one-hour sessions a week on massaging and caressing each other. This should be done in the privacy of the couple's bedroom, bathroom, or wherever they feel most comfortable.

The first sessions should consist of massaging nonsexual areas of the body, such as the back. As therapy proceeds, erotic and genital areas are gradually included, and, provided both partners feel comfortable, the emphasis shifts from the body alone to the body and genitals. During these early stages the couple should

not have intercourse, because an important part of sensate focus consists of each partner giving the other feedback on the response to being touched. This way the couple will improve the way they communicate verbally about sex and they will learn how to stimulate each other. Provided that the first stages of therapy go well, the couple eventually will move on to the problem areas concerning full intercourse.

What training do sex therapists have?
A sex therapist may have an M.D. in psychiatry, a Ph.D. in physiology, an M.S.W. in social work, or an M.S. in marital and family therapy. Unfortunately, not all people who call themselves sex therapists have received formal training. You can contact a local referral service of psychotherapists for the name of a qualified professional or ask your primary care physician to recommend someone.

WHAT YOU CAN DO AT HOME

One of the most important areas you can work on is establishing a comfortable and sensual environment for you and your partner.

A warm, gently lit room with fragrant candles and calming music, or bathing together in water that has

been scented with essential oils, such as ylang-ylang, can heighten the mood for sexual discovery and intimate physical contact.

Talk gently to one another and slowly caress each other until you are both fully at ease.

CREATING INTIMACY
A private and comfortable atmosphere can help you feel comfortable with your partner's body, and your own. You should be able to relax and focus on stimulating and caressing each other.

MALE PROBLEMS

The difficulties that men are most prone to include hormone-related problems like baldness, and conditions affecting the penis, testicles, and prostate gland.

Sperm count
Over the past 50 years, scientists have noticed a decline in the average male sperm count. They attribute this decline to increased levels of environmental pollution.

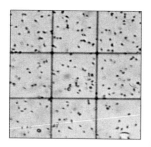

LOW SPERM COUNT
A poor sperm sample contains fewer than 20 million sperm per milliliter of semen.

HEALTHY SPERM COUNT
In a healthy fertile male, each milliliter of semen should contain at least 80 million sperm.

Men tend to have fewer urogenital tract infections than women. Male conditions, however, such as prostatitis and balanitis can be uncomfortable and may be transmitted to sexual partners. It is important that these ailments are promptly treated and that while under treatment, sensible precautions are observed during sexual intercourse.

BALANITIS

An inflammmation of the head of the penis, balanitis symptoms are soreness, swelling, and a discharge. It may be caused by injury, irritation, or a bacterial or yeast infection.

Infection can result from poor hygiene or from intercourse with an infected partner. For babies and children, it is commonly due to a tight foreskin or an allergic reaction to laundry detergent. Diabetic men are more susceptible to balanitis because the higher levels of sugar in their urine encourage bacteria to multiply.

See your doctor immediately if you suspect you have balanitis. If it's caused by an infection, use a condom during sexual intercourse because the infection can be passed back and forth between you and your partner.

Balanitis that arises from tight foreskin may need to be treated with circumcision. If balanitis has been caused by an allergy, use hypoallergenic condoms, change your laundry detergent, wear cotton underwear, and avoid perfumed soaps and bath products.

Recommended treatment for babies with balanitis includes frequent diaper changing and exposing the genital area to air.

Natural remedies for the relief of the symptoms of balanitis include naturopathy, hydrotherapy, and herbalism.

Naturopathy
To treat a yeast infection, reduce your intake of sugary foods and alcohol, and eat a cup of plain, live-culture yogurt every day.

Alternatively, you can take a teaspoon of acidophilus lactobacillus and bifidobacteria powder (available in health food stores) with water three times a day to help restore your body's balance of bacteria and yeast.

Hydrotherapy
Bathing the affected area in warm salt water three times a day may help soothe inflammation and promote healing.

Herbalism
Add five drops of essential oil of tea tree, which is both antibacterial and antifungal, to a basin of clean, warm water and bathe the penis regularly. After washing, dry the penis thoroughly and apply calendula cream to the irritated area to soothe inflammation.

LOW SPERM COUNT

The testes or testicles are paired oval glands that hang in a pouch outside the body and produce testosterone and sperm (at the rate of 100 million or more a day).

As many as one in six couples may suffer from infertility, and in about 30 percent of cases the cause is male infertility. This may be due to low sperm number, abnormal structure, or lack of motility. Raised temperature of the testes, environmental pollutants, alcohol, tobacco, and certain drugs can all cause low sperm count.

Conventional treatment for improving sperm count is a drug called clomiphene, which corrects hormonal imbalance. Problems with structure and motility are often more difficult to remedy. Avoiding tight underwear and pants may help.

Although low sperm count and infertility should be treated medically, herbalism, naturopathy, and relaxation may be useful.

Herbalism
Take 1 teaspoon of tincture of Siberian ginseng in a little water three times daily before meals, for up to 60 days. Avoid ginseng if you suffer from hypertension.

Naturopathy

Traditionally raw eggs or oysters were used to treat low sperm count. We now know that eggs contain vitamin B$_{12}$ and the quality protein needed to make sperm. Oysters contain zinc, which stimulates the formation of testosterone and aids erections and ejaculation. Scientific studies suggest that zinc tablets (220 milligrams), taken daily for at least four months, can improve sperm count. However, you should consult a doctor before taking zinc supplements.

The best approach is to eat a balanced diet of fresh fruits and vegetables—valuable sources of vitamin C; lean meat, poultry, eggs, and shellfish for vitamin B$_{12}$; wheat germ, nuts, seeds, and vegetable oils—sources of vitamin E; and oysters, liver, wheat germ, and sunflower or pumpkin seeds for zinc. Vitamin C and vitamin B$_{12}$ supplements may also help.

Avoid alcohol completely—it may be harmful to the male reproductive system—and abstain from tobacco and caffeine.

Relaxation

If your energy reserves are depleted by a hectic schedule or chronic stress, your body may close down unnecessary processes, one of which could be sperm production. Give yourself time during the day to relieve stress with relaxation techniques (see page 114).

PROSTATITIS

The prostate gland is located beneath the bladder encircling the urethra—the tube through which urine and semen are expelled. The prostate gland produces secretions that form part of the seminal fluid that is released during ejaculation.

Infection or inflammation of the gland—prostatitis—may be a result of a sexually transmitted infection spreading from the urethra, although this is not always the case. The symptoms of prostatitis are frequent, painful urination, possibly with blood in the urine; pain on ejaculation; fever; lower back pain; abdominal pain; and sometimes a tender, enlarged prostate. You should see your doctor if you have any of these symptoms; they can also denote other serious conditions, all of which require medical attention.

The conventional treatment for prostatitis is bed rest, painkillers, and antibiotics, but herbalism, naturopathy, and hydrotherapy may give additional help by strengthening the immune system and relieving symptoms.

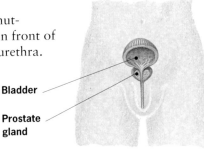

PROSTATE GLAND

The prostate gland is a chestnut-shaped, solid organ that sits in front of the rectum, surrounding the urethra.

PROSTATE INFECTION
This can lead to painful symptoms, including urinary problems, which should be treated by a doctor.

Bladder

Prostate gland

Herbalism

A standard infusion of equal parts of meadowsweet, buchu, and corn silk has diuretic and antiseptic properties. Drink several times a day as needed. Echinacea may also help. Take $\frac{1}{2}$ teaspoon of tincture or one 500-milligram capsule three times daily.

Naturopathy

Naturopaths are likely to recommend zinc for prostatitis. Watercress, oysters, herring, oatmeal, and sunflower and pumpkin seeds are all good sources of zinc, but you can also take it as a supplement: 30 milligrams daily is recommended. Consult a doctor before taking zinc supplements.

Hydrotherapy

Sitz baths (see page 21) can increase circulation and relax muscles in the pelvic area around the prostate. Sit for three minutes in hot water, and 30 seconds in cold water. Repeat three times, finishing with the cold bath. Perform daily, but be sure to keep the rest of your body covered to avoid chills.

ENLARGED PROSTATE

Due to hormonal changes associated with aging, about 50 percent of males by age 60 have a prostate gland that is enlarged enough to cause some discomfort. The sufferer experiences the need to urinate frequently, to the extent that sleep may be interrupted more than twice every night. Difficulties with passing urine are common; they include a weakened flow and interruption and dribbling of urine. Eventually the bladder may not be able to empty, causing abdominal swelling and pain. See your doctor if you develop these symptoms.

Conventional treatment includes prescription drugs that improve bladder emptying, but if an enlarged prostate causes severe symptoms, it may be partially removed. A new technique involves sending a low-

ECHINACEA CAPSULES
Widely recommended by herbalists as a remedy for infections, echinacea (in capsule or tincture form) may relieve the symptoms of prostatitis.

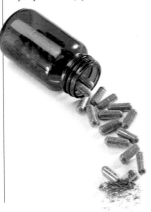

power burst of electrical energy through the urethra to shrink part of the prostate—an outpatient procedure. Herbalism, naturopathy, and exercise can be used as adjuncts to conventional medical treatments.

Herbalism

Stinging nettle root in capsule or tablet form may relieve the urinary symptoms associated with an enlarged prostate gland. You can also make a standard decoction of the herb and drink it three times a day between meals over a period of two months. An herbalist may recommend a tincture of saw palmetto berries to help clear the gland of androgens (male sex hormones) and relieve symptoms of prostate enlargement. Recent tests have shown it to be quite effective, but it should be taken under a doctor's supervision, as it may interact with prescription drugs.

Naturopathy

Taken daily, the following remedies may help minimize symptoms of an enlarged prostate: 50 to 80 milligrams of zinc (consult a doctor before taking zinc supplements), 800 international units of vitamin E (consult a doctor before taking vitamin E if you have heart disease or hypertension), and a tablespoon of corn or safflower oil for polyunsaturated fats.

Eat a balanced diet with lots of fresh fruits and vegetables and cut down on red meat and foods that are high in cholesterol. Some waste products of cholesterol accumulate in the prostate gland. For this reason a low-fat, low-cholesterol diet may help ease the symptoms of an enlarged prostate.

Eat tofu and other soybean products. It's believed that these may protect the prostate gland from high levels of dihydrotestosterone, a male hormone that stimulates the overgrowth of prostate tissue.

Some foods contain particularly therapeutic combinations of nutrients—pumpkin seeds, for example. They have essential fatty acids and zinc, and an active compound called curcurbitin. Research in Sweden has shown that curcurbitin improves urinary flow and reduces nighttime urination. Several European countries now market a medication based on curcurbitin.

Exercise

Walking massages the prostate, toning the muscles of that area, and increasing blood circulation. Try to take an hour-long walk each day. Kegel exercises (see page 143) can also help strengthen these muscles.

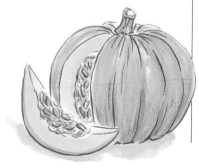

PUMPKIN SEEDS
A cup of pumpkin seeds eaten every day is a folk remedy for enlarged prostate. They may alleviate symptoms due to their diuretic properties that increase the flow of urine.

HAIR LOSS AND BALDNESS

Alopecia, commonly known as hair loss or baldness, may result from hormonal changes, especially those linked to aging. Alopecia may be hereditary. It can affect men, and occasionally women, of any age. If it is hereditary, alopecia tends to follow a certain pattern for men, with the normal hair at the temples and on the crown being affected first and replaced with a fine down. A nonhereditary, temporary thinning or major loss of hair can be the result of stress, prolonged illness, nutritional deficiencies, or chemotherapy.

Conventional treatment includes restoring or replacing hair. Drugs may be rubbed into the scalp or injected under the scalp. The latter usually has only short-term effects. Alternatively, hair roots from other areas of the body can be transplanted to the head (this is a lengthy and expensive procedure).

Therapies such as herbalism and naturopathy may improve the health of the scalp and hair and encourage growth.

Herbalism

An herbalist can help identify the underlying causes of hair loss and prescribe herbs to support the general health of the body. Rosemary and lavender promote circulation to the scalp, stimulate the roots, and help condition the hair.

Massage oil of rosemary into the scalp before shampooing (see page 59). Follow with an herbal conditioning rinse consisting of 2 tablespoons each of dried lavender, rosemary, and nettle, steeped in 32 fluid ounces (1 quart) of boiling water for at least 30 minutes. Add 1 tablespoon of cider vinegar and pour over the hair, then rinse thoroughly. For best effects, repeat this procedure for the next 20 times that you shampoo.

Naturopathy

Try to eat at least five servings of fresh fruits and vegetables (especially green peppers, broccoli, and watercress) a day. Fish, eggs, meat, wheat germ, and legumes should be your main sources of protein. These foods contain not only appreciable levels of protein but also vitamins C, E, and B, iron, and zinc—all essential for healthy hair.

Taking vitamin B complex daily can increase the blood supply to the scalp and nourish the nervous system; 50 milligrams of zinc taken daily may help hair growth, although the effects may take some time. Consult a doctor before taking zinc supplements.

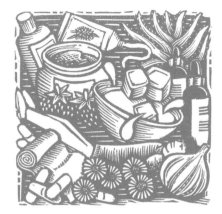

CHAPTER 11

ACCIDENTS AND INJURIES

Natural remedies are ideal for treating
sprains, strains, cuts, stings, bites, and bruises.
In the case of minor accidents, it is very easy to
apply a soothing compress or massage a painful
joint. Many of the items you will need for a natural
first-aid kit can be found in the garden or
the kitchen cupboard at home.

EVERYDAY INJURIES

Minor injuries don't usually cause long-term health problems, as long as they are treated properly. A combination of first aid and natural remedies can help relieve pain and speed recovery.

In many cases, the application of hot and cold compresses and herbal ointments to slight injuries can help to reduce the chances of lengthy periods of recuperation, infection, or scarring.

SPRAINS AND STRAINS

Although some regard the terms "strain" and "sprain" as synonymous, it is more accurate to consider wrenched, torn, or overstretched muscles as strains, and more extensive injuries to the ligaments around a joint as sprains.

The symptoms of a strain may include muscle stiffness, bruising, and swelling, and the area may be either tender to the touch or quite painful. If the suspected strain is actually a ruptured muscle, then the surrounding muscles may pull the injured tissues apart and surgery may be necessary.

A sprain, on the other hand, is clearly characterized by swelling, bruising, and sharp pain around the affected joint. It usually is painful to move the joint and to bear weight on it. If the sprain is very severe, it will be almost impossible to use the affected joint for weeks or months. The symptoms of a severe sprain may mimic those of a fracture; an X-ray may be necessary to clear up doubt. Some sprains require such medical treatment as long-term immobilization or, in the most serious cases, surgery to repair the torn ligaments.

Muscles are richly supplied with blood vessels that aid the body's healing processes so that they will recover from minor strains within a few days. Ligaments, however, recover very slowly because they are fibrous and thick and have a poor blood supply. If severely injured, they can be more painful and slower to heal than broken bones.

After first aid has been applied, anti-inflammatory drugs or painkillers may help. Natural therapies for sprains and strains include homeopathy, acupressure, massage, and herbalism to relieve immediate pain, and osteopathy to ease long-term discomfort.

For pain that lasts more than a few days or does not respond to natural or conventional first aid, see your doctor. Your injury should be properly diagnosed in case there has been extensive tissue damage.

Standard first aid

Immediately apply an ice pack (or a bag of frozen vegetables as an emergency substitute) to reduce the pain and swelling. Raise and support the injured joint or muscle and immobilize it with elastic bandages to minimize swelling and discomfort.

Homeopathy

Arnica For pain within the first 24 hours. You can also apply arnica cream or ointment to the injured area.

Ruta graveolens For the long-term recovery of ligament and tendon injury.

Ledum For pain associated with coldness but relieved by cold applications.

Rhus toxicodendron For joint stiffness or pain that improves with movement.

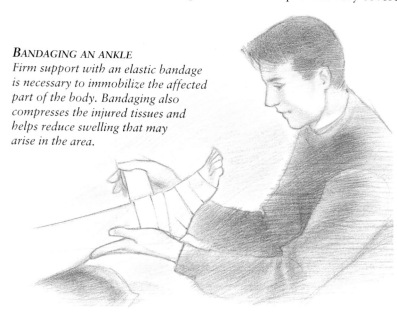

BANDAGING AN ANKLE
Firm support with an elastic bandage is necessary to immobilize the affected part of the body. Bandaging also compresses the injured tissues and helps reduce swelling that may arise in the area.

Acupressure
Massage GB 34 and TB 5 for a few minutes twice daily. Apply pressure to both arms and both legs. Acupuncture may also help.

Massage
The most effective stroke is effleurage—light kneading and stroking toward the heart. Start several inches away from the injury and then work toward it. This will help to improve circulation and drain built-up fluid.

Herbalism
A poultice made with comfrey leaves may be applied to a swollen, injured joint. Bruise the leaves with a rolling pin and place them in a dressing of gauze or muslin. The leaves may cause irritation, so do not put them directly on the skin.

Osteopathy
Many practitioners use soft tissue treatments, such as neuromuscular technique, which improves the circulation to the sprained joint and helps the rehabilitation of old sprains and strains by dispersing any fibrous thickening. Muscle energy techniques work gently to stretch fibers that may antagonize the damaged ones. Such techniques produce relaxation and rebalance the tension of the injured muscles.

BRUISES
A bruise occurs when capillaries that lie beneath the surface of the skin are damaged by a blow or severe pressure, allowing blood to diffuse into the tissues. Although some people bruise more easily than others, spontaneous bruising (occurring without obvious injury or from light pressure only) may result from nutritional deficiencies or blood disorders. If you bruise easily, see your doctor.

Standard first aid
Either place cold compresses or run cold water on the injured area. Do not apply ice directly to the skin because this may damage small blood vessels.

Herbalism
As long as the skin is not broken, arnica cream may be applied to the bruise twice every day until it is completely healed. Arnica can also be taken as a homeopathic remedy. Alternatively, you can use tincture of witch hazel mixed with water to make a cold compress. Add 1 teaspoon of the tincture to every teaspoon of water.

Naturopathy
If you bruise easily, eat a diet rich in foods containing antioxidants, such as dark green, orange, and yellow vegetables and fruits. Cauliflower, broccoli, and cabbage are rich in flavone compounds, which are thought to protect the blood vessels and promote healing. Plain live-culture yogurt may promote the bacteria that help synthesize vitamin K in the gut. Vitamin K helps to prevent blood vessel fragility. You can also drink pineapple juice for its bromelaine content, an enzyme that is thought to thin clotted blood.

CUTS AND ABRASIONS
The skin is your body's protection against the external environment. A cut or abrasion breaches that defense and, although your body is equipped to heal itself quickly and

Acupressure for strains

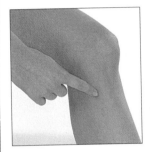

PRESSURE POINT GB 34
This is located on the outer surface of the knee joint below the head of the fibula bone, between the tendons.

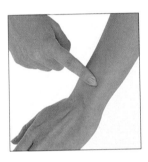

PRESSURE POINT TB 5
This point is on the outer forearm, three finger widths above the wrist crease between the bones.

HERBAL TREATMENT FOR CUTS AND ABRASIONS

Minor injuries can be treated with herbal preparations. Tea tree and calendula (marigold) are thought to have antiseptic properties whereas comfrey ointment may help to speed healing by encouraging cell growth. To reduce the risk of infection, wounds should be cleaned with water before remedies are applied to the skin.

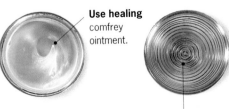

Use healing comfrey ointment.

Add tea tree oil to water for cleaning a wound.

HERBAL OINTMENT AND OIL
An application of comfrey ointment and tea tree oil may help to heal minor cuts and abrasions.

CALENDULA CREAM
This popular remedy, which is also called marigold cream, can be applied to minor injuries that break the skin.

Calendula cream helps prevent infection.

Protect yourself against insect bites and stings using the following measures:

▶ *Wear light-colored, loose clothing that covers your arms and legs.*

▶ *Use screens or nets in bedrooms whenever you are staying in areas where mosquitoes and other biting insects are likely to attack.*

▶ *Avoid using perfumes and aftershave lotions that might attract insects.*

▶ *Avoid sugar and other sweet foods in the diet. Excessive sugar in the blood may attract insects. It also increases the level of histamine in the blood, which promotes inflammatory reactions to bites and stings.*

▶ *Vitamin B$_1$ (100 milligrams three times a day) and garlic tablets (2 or 3 tablets daily) are reputed to have a deterrent effect when taken regularly.*

▶ *Natural insect repellents include citronella and eucalyptus essential oils. These can be used in oil burners.*

efficiently, you should still take steps to protect against infection. Proper cleansing of cuts and abrasions and adequate protection against tetanus are important. After first-aid measures have been applied, herbalism and homeopathy may help.

Standard first aid
If the wound contains dirt, cleanse it gently with plenty of water. If there is any foreign material in the wound that cannot be washed away, see a doctor. Otherwise, raise the wound above the level of the victim's head to reduce bleeding. If the wound is on the leg or foot, have the victim lie on the floor and prop the wounded limb on a raised surface. Provided there is no danger of excessive blood loss, allow the wound to bleed for a few minutes to help cleanse it. Stanch bleeding with a sterile dressing, drawing the sides of the wound together before covering. If bleeding is severe or the wound is deep, apply firm pressure to the wound with clean gauze and seek medical attention immediately. If the wound was caused by a garden implement or a dirty or rusty object, seek immediate medical advice and antitetanus treatment.

Herbalism
Cleanse the wound with water to which has been added a few drops of calendula (marigold) tincture or hypercal—a mixture of hypericum and calendula. Herbalists believe that calendula promotes healing and is mildly antiseptic. Treat minor wounds with a light application of calendula cream and cover with a sterile dressing.

Homeopathy
Hypericum For dirt entering the wound or a wound caused by a rusty or dirty object.
Ledum For pain or for wounds caused by sharp objects.

INSECT BITES AND STINGS
A wide variety of crawling or flying creatures can cause discomfort to humans through bites and stings that penetrate the skin. Many of these creatures, such as black flies, mosquitoes, and horseflies, will bite without warning at the first opportunity. Others, such as wasps and bees, will sting only when provoked or disturbed.

Occasionally insect bites become infected, causing pain, tenderness, swelling, and possibly a yellow-green discharge of pus. Some people have severe reactions to insect stings, particularly if they already have high blood

levels of histamine, a chemical released by the body during an allergic reaction. They may suffer swelling, impaired breathing, severe itching, dizziness, vomiting, and a rapid pulse. This is anaphylactic shock, which requires injections of epinephrine.

Natural remedies for bites and stings include herbalism, homeopathy, naturopathy, and folk remedies.

Standard first aid
If the stinger is left in the skin, remove it and any venom sac, by gently scraping with a card, knife, or fingernail; do not use tweezers. Apply a cold compress to relieve discomfort. For stings in the mouth, see a doctor or go to a hospital immediately. For bites, clean and apply calamine lotion for itching, and an antibiotic ointment if an infection develops.

Herbalism
Bruise fresh plantain leaves and apply them directly to bites and stings. *Aloe vera* can also be soothing—use either a prepared ointment or juice taken directly from the leaves.

Homeopathy
Ledum For most bites or stings.
Apis mellifica For alleviating the pain of many stings, especially beestings.

Naturopathy
Practitioners recommend vitamin C to reduce inflammation and counteract high levels of histamine in the blood. The oil from a capsule of vitamin E applied directly to the sting may promote recovery.

FOLK REMEDIES FOR STINGS

Hold the cut surface of an onion in place over the sting, or bind it with a handkerchief or elastic bandage, and keep it on for several hours.

Alternatively, apply a compress made with apple cider vinegar or a poultice made with bicarbonate of soda or simple unperfumed soap.

RAW ONION REMEDY
Apply a slice of raw onion to bee and wasp stings to reduce the irritation.

OTHER INJURIES

Natural remedies can help relieve pain or speed recovery, but severe injuries should always be treated first by a qualified health care professional.

Serious injuries, such as bone fractures, severe loss of blood, loss of consciousness, sudden breathing problems, head injuries, and any injuries that result in loss of sight, hearing, or feeling in any part of the body are medical emergencies. They must be treated immediately with conventional medical care to ensure that the victim's recovery is as complete and problem-free as possible.

Although these injuries are not covered here, natural remedies can be used after the initial conventional medical treatment to help speed recovery, by aiding the healing process and strengthening the body.

Natural remedies and standard first-aid measures can be used together to treat the symptoms of mild cases of sunburn, heat exhaustion, burns, and accidental poisoning.

SUNBURN

The effects of overexposure to the sun may not become apparent for up to 24 hours after exposure. In the majority of cases there will be redness with burning pain, itching, or irritation of the affected areas, which may lead to blisters. Very severe sunburn may be accompanied by chills, fever, shock, and dehydration—the symptoms of heatstroke or sunstroke—and should be treated as a medical emergency (see page 155).

Herbalism, aromatherapy, homeopathy, and acupressure may provide symptom relief from sunburn, but staying out of direct sunlight is best.

Standard first aid

Apply compresses to the body with towels soaked in cold water, or take a cold shower. A cool or tepid bath with either 2 tablespoons of cider vinegar or 2 tablespoons of bicarbonate of soda added to it may be soothing. You should also apply calamine lotion to the affected areas. Painkillers, such as aspirin or acetaminophen, may help.

If you are badly sunburned, you may be dehydrated. Until symptoms ease, drink eight glasses of water a day. Avoid alcohol.

Herbalism

Aloe vera soothes and heals burns. Apply an ointment prepared from the plant or use the juice from the leaf. Hypercal lotion or cream (a mixture of hypericum and calendula) may encourage healing.

Aromatherapy

Add five drops of lavender essential oil to a small glass of almond oil and apply to the affected area.

Homeopathy

Urtica urens For prickly itching and burning sensations.

Rhus toxicodendron For severe blistering.

Acupressure

Apply gentle kneading pressure to a point known as Chao-chang (see illustration at right). Press both thumbs, using your finger or a rounded pen top.

PREVENTING SUNBURN

Repeated exposure to the sun over many years leads to dry, prematurely wrinkled skin and an increased risk of skin cancer. To limit the extent of the damage, try to avoid exposure to the sun between 10 A.M. and 3 P.M. and always wear protective clothing, such as hats and closely woven T-shirts (this is especially important when you are exposed to reflected light while swimming, walking, or sailing). Also, remember that wind can intensify burning, even though you may feel cool. Always apply a sunscreen with a sun protection factor (SPF) of 15 or greater, particularly to your shoulders, face, and chest. Reapply sunscreen regularly, especially after swimming.

Acupressure for sunburn

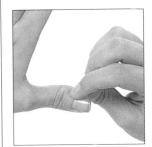

PRESSURE POINT CHAO-CHANG
This point does not lie on the conventional meridian system. It is located just below the corner of the thumbnail on the side closer to the first finger. Treat both of the thumbs.

Relieving Sunburn with

Home Remedies

There are several handy remedies for sunburn that you may already have in your kitchen cupboard or elsewhere in your home. Preparation of these treatments is simple, and their pain-relieving properties are safe and effective.

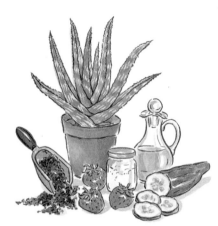

COOLING APPLICATIONS
Household staples such as tea, vinegar, bicarbonate of soda, strawberries, and cucumber can help to relieve sunburn. Aloe vera is also useful.

A cool bath or shower is the best way to relieve the pain of sunburn. You can increase the soothing effects of a bath by adding vinegar, bicarbonate of soda, or finely ground oatmeal to the water. Alternatively, make a compress or poultice using any of the above, and apply it to your skin.

A weak infusion of black tea, allowed to cool, can be used as a wash to ease sunburned skin.

Like tea, strawberries contain astringent tannins that may help to relieve sunburn. Spread the crushed fruit on the skin or apply as a poultice.

If you are suffering from sunburn on your face, particularly around your eyes, place a slice of peeled cucumber over each eye. Leave in place for approximately 15 minutes. This should ease the burning of the sensitive skin in this area.

TREATING SUNBURN WITH *ALOE VERA*

The fresh juice obtained from a split *Aloe vera* leaf is a well-accepted, widely used remedy for sunburn. The cooling and soothing properties of *Aloe vera* juice quickly help to ease the stinging pain of a burn, and its moisturizing action deeply penetrates the layers of the skin and works to prevent the peeling that often follows sunburn.

Although *Aloe vera* is available commercially in ointment form, the plant is easy to cultivate, and growing your own *Aloe vera* ensures that you have a ready source of the purest and freshest juice. Store-bought ointments are adequate for treating sunburn, but the purer the remedy the more effective are its healing properties.

APPLYING THE JUICE
When you have extracted enough juice, apply it directly to your skin, gently smoothing it over the affected areas.

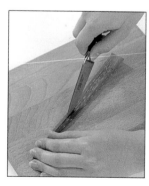

CUTTING A LEAF
Remove one leaf and, using a sharp knife, make a straight incision on one side, along its entire length.

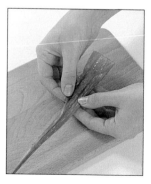

OPENING IT
Use your fingers to open the leaf so that the whole of the inside of the leaf is exposed.

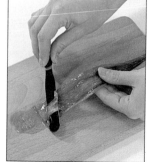

EXTRACTING THE JUICE
Using a dinner knife or spoon, carefully scrape out the inside of the leaf onto a flat, nonabsorbent surface.

HEAT EXHAUSTION AND HEATSTROKE

Heat exhaustion is caused by dehydration, usually the result of sweating heavily and not consuming adequate replacement fluids. Warning signs include fatigue, weakness, and feelings of anxiety, along with drenching sweat. As the condition worsens, blood pressure drops, the pulse slows, and the skin becomes pale and clammy. The person could be confused and might faint.

Heatstroke develops when the body's ability to cool itself by sweating fails during very hot, humid weather. It can quickly lead to a fever of 104°F or higher. Symptoms include hot, dry skin; a rapid pulse; fast, shallow breathing; confusion; and unconsciousness or convulsions. Heatstroke is potentially life threatening, and immediate medical attention should be sought.

To avoid heat exhaustion and heatstroke, limit the time you spend in the sun, and gradually build up your exposure to heat over a two-week period. Avoid strenuous outdoor exercise and wear light, loose clothing and a hat or scarf for protection from the sun. Drink plenty of fluids, particularly water, but avoid alcohol and caffeine.

If the symptoms of heat exhaustion or heatstroke develop, apply standard first-aid measures and seek medical attention. Naturopathy and homeopathy may aid rehydration and recuperation. Hydrotherapy can also be helpful.

Standard first aid

For heat exhaustion, move the sufferer to cool surroundings and help him or her to lie down. Raise the legs above the level of the head and prevent dehydration by helping the person to sip a cool, weak salt solution. Consult a doctor as soon as possible to rule out the possibility of heatstroke.

Seek immediate emergency medical treatment for anyone suspected of suffering from heatstroke. In the meantime, move the victim to cool surroundings and help him or her to lie down. Raise the feet so that they are higher than the rest of the body—this will improve blood flow from the legs to the upper body. Remove any clothing and either sponge the entire body with cool water, or wrap the person in sheets soaked in water. Fan the victim by hand or with an electric fan. When the body temperature falls to 100°F, stop sponging, or replace the wet sheets with dry ones, but continue to fan.

Naturopathy

Prevent symptoms of heatstroke by drinking plenty of water. If you think you are developing heat exhaustion, drink a very dilute salt and sugar solution (¼ teaspoon of each in a pint of water).

While recovering from heatstroke or exhaustion, drink only fruit juices or water until you are feeling better. Then start to eat foods such as fruit salads and steamed vegetables. Avoid all stimulants, such as tea, coffee, and alcohol, for at least a day or two.

Homeopathy

Glonoine For throbbing headache accompanied by giddiness.

Belladonna For throbbing headache made worse by lying down.

Gelsemium For pain at the nape of the neck, with flushed face and hot dry skin.

Hydrotherapy

Frequent cool showers or baths during very hot weather can help prevent heat exhaustion or heatstroke. Be especially careful when swimming; although your body may feel cool, your head is still exposed to the sun and reflected sunlight can be intense.

BURNS

Whether caused by exposure to heat, chemicals, or electricity, burns are classified according to severity. First-degree burns are the mildest, involving the top layers of skin,

---

FIRST AID FOR BURNS

Immediately rinse the burn under cold running water or immerse it in cold water. If you do not have a sterile dressing, cover the burn with a plastic bag or plastic wrap as a temporary measure.

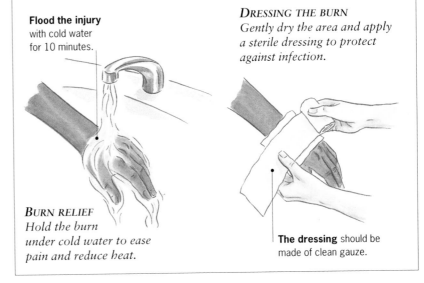

Flood the injury with cold water for 10 minutes.

DRESSING THE BURN
Gently dry the area and apply a sterile dressing to protect against infection.

BURN RELIEF
Hold the burn under cold water to ease pain and reduce heat.

The dressing should be made of clean gauze.

Acupressure for poisoning

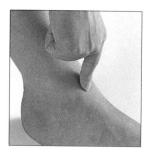

PRESSURE POINT ST 41
This point is on the front of the ankle joint in the depression between the two tendons.

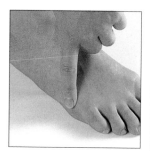

PRESSURE POINT BL 65
This can be located on the outer edge of the foot in the depression behind the joint at the base of the little toe.

resulting in redness and pain. Second-degree burns extend beneath the surface layer and require medical treatment. They leave the skin looking raw and blistered. Third-degree burns are the most severe; the skin may be blackened and damage extends usually below the skin to affect nerves, blood vessels, even muscles and bone. With anything but the mildest of superficial burns, it is vital to seek medical attention. Note that therapies such as herbalism, homeopathy, aromatherapy, and folk remedies are recommended for minor burns only.

Standard first aid
Hold the injured part of the body under cold running water for about 10 minutes and then remove any jewelery or clothes from the affected area. Cover the burn with a sterile dressing—avoid using fluffy material that might adhere to the burned skin. Do not apply butter to a burn. Be careful not to break any blisters or interfere in any way with the burned area.

Herbalism
Add a few drops of calendula tincture to cold water and use the solution to make a compress. Alternatively, try adding 1 teaspoon of tincture of stinging nettle to cold water and apply as a compress using a soaked pad of gauze. Replace the compress every two to three hours.

Aloe vera juice or ointment or calendula cream can be applied directly to mild burns after the heat and pain have been taken out of the burn with cold water.

Homeopathy
Urtica urens For relief from the pain and discomfort of a burn.
Causticum For burns with pain, restlessness, and blisters.
Aconite For sharp, stabbing pain.

Aromatherapy
Essential oil of lavender may be applied to mild burns once symptoms have subsided. Add 5 drops to ½ cup of almond oil and apply twice a day.

Folk remedies
Honey is used to prevent infection and promote healing of minor burns. A dressing of honey may be applied after standard first-aid measures have taken effect.

ACCIDENTAL POISONING
Stomach irritation and nausea, usually followed by cramping, vomiting, and possibly diarrhea, are the most common symptoms of poisoning. In severe cases, the heart, brain, lungs, and kidneys may be involved and result in stupor, a fluctuating pulse rate, and changes in urinary output. If you suspect poisoning, treat it as a medical emergency—seek immediate help by calling your local poison control center, emergency medical services, or doctor.

Collect any bottles, containers, foodstuffs, and even samples of vomit that may help to identify the poison. Take them with you to show the doctor.

Acupressure can be used while waiting for medical assistance. Herbalism and homeopathy, on the other hand, may help, but you should practice them only after the victim has received conventional medical care.

Standard first aid
Stay with the victim and place him or her in a position that will keep the airways clear of vomit. Do not give anything to eat or drink or any substance that may encourage vomiting—the regurgitation of a caustic substance can cause further damage. Seek medical help immediately.

Acupressure
For vomiting and perspiration, apply pressure for one to two minutes to point LI 4 (see page 68). This is on the fleshy tissue in the angle between the thumb and first finger (avoid LI 4 during pregnancy). For violent abdominal pain, massage St 41. For burning sensations in the mouth or throat, apply steady pressure for a few minutes to Bl 65.

Herbalism
After you have consulted your doctor and the immediate symptoms of poisoning have abated, try slippery elm bark. This will help by providing a protective coating and soothing the inflamed surfaces in the stomach and intestines. Mix 1 heaping teaspoon of slippery elm bark powder with a little honey, then slowly add warm water or milk to make a consistency that is acceptable for drinking or eating with a spoon. It should be taken before each meal for several days following the poisoning.

Homeopathy
Aconite For the person who is anxious, restless, or fearful.
Arnica For the patient who is sleepy and in a state of shock.
Veratum album For vomiting and diarrhea with profuse cold sweating.
Arsenicum album For diarrhea with a burning stomach, anxiety, and chills.

INDEX

158

ACKNOWLEDGMENTS

Carroll & Brown Limited
would like to thank
Ellen Dupont
Juliette Kando
Sue Mimms

Mark Blumenthal
Executive Director, American
Botanical Council, Editor,
Herbalgram, Austin, TX

Joseph E. Keaney, Principal of the Irish
School of Ethical and Analytical
Hypnotherapy, Ireland

The Water Monopoly, London

Photograph sources
8 Malcolm Crowthers
13 Rex Features
16 Bibliotheque Nationale,
Paris/Bridgeman Art Library
20 Ronald Sheridan/Ancient Art and
Architecture Collection
22 The Bach Centre
23 The Charles Walker
Collection/Images Colour Library
24 Image Bank/Gio Barto
27 Zefa
28 John Walmsley
30 Tony Stone Images
31 Mary Evans Picture Library
32 By permission of the British
Library, London
57 Melanie Friend/Hutchison Library
65 British Library, London/Bridgeman
Art Library
68 A.B. Dowsett/SPL
71 Tony Stone Images
88 BSIP, Stephant/SPL
100 RelaxPlus by Ultramind Limited
120 Tony Stone Images
125 Image Bank/William Sallaz
140 Prof. P. Motta/Dept. of
Anatomy/University 'La Sapienza',
Rome/SPL
146 Nurture

Illustrators
Louise Boulton
Joanna Cameron
John Geary
Frances Lloyd
Vanessa Luff
Melanie Northover
Christine Pilsworth
Ann Winterbotham
Angela Wood

Charts
Nick Roland

Photographic assistance
Nick Allen
Sid Sideris

Picture researcher
Sandra Schneider

Food preparation
Maddalena Bastianelli

Index
Madeline Weston

Note
Imperial measures are given throughout
except when calculating measures of
nutrients, which are given in metric.